COLIC SOLVED

COLIC
SOLVED

THE ESSENTIAL GUIDE
TO INFANT REFLUX AND THE
CARE OF YOUR CRYING,
DIFFICULT-TO-SOOTHE BABY

Bryan Vartabedian, M.D.

BALLANTINE BOOKS / NEW YORK

A Ballantine Books Trade Paperback Original

Copyright © 2007 by Bryan Vartabedian, M.D.

Published in the United States by Ballantine Books, an imprint of The Random House Publishing Group, a division of Random House, Inc., New York.

BALLANTINE and colophon are registered trademarks of Random House, Inc.

ISBN 978-0-345-49068-1

LIBRARY OF CONGRESS CATALOGING-IN-PUBLICATION DATA
Vartabedian, Bryan S.
Colic solved : the essential guide to infant reflux and the care of your crying, difficult-to-soothe baby / Bryan Vartabedian.
p. cm.
Includes index.
ISBN 978-0-345-49068-1
1. Colic.   I. Title.
RJ267.V37 2007   618.92'09755—dc22   2006042877

Printed in the United States of America

www.ballantinebooks.com

2 4 6 8 9 7 5 3

Illustrations by Briar Lee Mitchell

Book design by Casey Hampton

For Deidre

ACKNOWLEDGMENTS

Colic Solved would never have come to be without the help of several people. Kevan Lyon of the Sandra Dijkstra Literary Agency recognized the potential hidden in this project and put it in the right hands. Nancy Miller, my editor at Ballantine/ Random House, recognized that crying babies need a voice and jumped on this project the moment she laid eyes on it. Alison Simmons, Wendy Rosenfeld, and Marna Lewis provided valuable maternal input and encouraged this project from its earliest stages. I thank Briar Lee Mitchell for her beautiful illustrations. Laura Miller, R.N., at the Texas Children's Health Center—The Woodlands, compulsively tended to my parent phone calls and schedule so that this book could be completed. Dr. Craig Jensen provided sharp-witted technical review. This book never would have made it without my frontline editor, wife, and one-woman focus group, Deidre, who selflessly allowed me to isolate myself and write. Finally, I credit my colleagues past and present at Texas Children's Hospital and beyond who have dedicated themselves to the advancement of pediatric digestive disease and created the standards and studies that keep our children healthy and happy.

CONTENTS

INTRODUCTION

Perhaps you've heard about it but never thought it would happen to you. You are new parents to a miserable, inconsolable newborn with intractable screaming who can't sleep and can barely feed. Sleepless, selfless nights are spent in desperation for just a few moments of peace that don't seem to ever come. Days seem to run into one another. It's misery for you and your baby. You feel helpless.

While you hold out hope that your pediatrician holds the key, you get the feeling after your first visit that perhaps you shouldn't be so concerned. Another visit, two formulas, and three phone calls later, you definitely get the feeling that you've overstayed your welcome. And while the health care providers never quite come out and say it, you can almost hear "We've done all we can do." Through all of this there's a part of you that feels like a bad parent who's either not doing something right or who can't cope with something that all parents are supposed to cope with. You never signed up for this.

So what is it and what can you do? Why is your baby the way she is? And why can't she just be happy like the baby next door? This is what *Colic Solved* is about. It offers new answers to these questions and provides parents with medically proven solutions that pediatric gastroenterologists recommend. The answers in the following pages have come through the advancements in medical technology that have occurred since the time when a doctor's only answer to a baby's screaming was "colic." Keep in mind that *colic* was defined during an era when doctors were seen posing in cigarette ads. But times have changed, and the way that pediatricians see babies has changed. Yet even today, thousands of irritable babies with treatable problems are overlooked and their conditions are labeled as everything from "colic" to "irresponsible parenting." The pages ahead aim to help you understand our most current approach to the miserable baby. Beyond understanding, *Colic Solved* will empower you to advocate for your baby.

I suggest in *Colic Solved* that there isn't such a thing as colic. Colic is instead a well-orchestrated five-letter defense mechanism for doctors who are either outdated, outwitted, or just plain out of ideas. We now know that children with the type of irritability described as colic most likely suffer with either reflux or milk protein hypersensitivity. Books such as *The Happiest Baby on the Block* and *Secrets of the Baby Whisperer* simply perpetuate the concept that the only thing wrong is a parent who doesn't know how to swaddle properly or make the right shushing noises. *Colic Solved* is the ultimate validation for the parent of the irritable baby.

Our experience and medical research tell us that the fussy baby is fussy for a reason, and *Colic Solved* will help those parents looking for answers. While *Colic Solved* doesn't intend to suggest that there aren't high-need babies or those with sensitive nervous systems, it is here to introduce the idea that something physical may in fact be wrong. This book will serve as a starting point for understanding that the answer to a baby's crying lies not in a rigid schedule or the proper shushing sound but rather in the belief that a baby's pain is treatable and real.

Colic Solved will help you understand if your baby is suffering with one of the most common causes of infant irritability, acid reflux. Once thought to be nonexistent in children, acid reflux disease in children is being recognized more frequently, and children are getting help. Finally there's something that can be done besides make shushing noises.

Over the months that I wrote *Colic Solved*, I consulted a number of my colleagues on some of the fuzzier issues of infant reflux and confirmed what my grandfather always told me: There's more than one way to skin a cat. Or in this case, there's more than one way to handle the baby who screams all the time.

Some of my colleagues think I make too much out of reflux; others think I haven't said enough. There are those who may disagree with my opinion of the role of reflux in infant irritability, but the fact is, its recognition and treatment works with most babies. My real goal in this book is twofold: (1) to get tired parents asking questions and (2) to provide them with the best answers and solutions possible.

Given some of the varying styles of managing reflux, the North American Society of Pediatric Gastroenterology, Hepatology, and Nutrition (or NASPGHAN, the formal organization of pediatric tummy doctors) got together in 2001 to create a consensus on the management of infant and childhood reflux. The result was a monumental position paper created for pediatricians and other pediatric specialists to help guide them in the diagnosis and treatment of childhood reflux. It has created a framework from which to work for those less experienced with reflux disease. But like anything else created by a committee, it has its strengths and weaknesses when it comes down to the nuts and bolts of "what to do" with a baby who gives as much as she receives.

While I've done my best to embody the spirit and soul of the NASPGHAN guidelines in these pages, I have to admit that this book is peppered with my stubborn opinions that have been molded over the past several years by thousands of screaming babies, griping parents, and burping toddlers. I have tried to make it clear when my opinion deviates from that of my colleagues who worked hard to create the often-quoted NASPGHAN guidelines. Some of what you read will be straight party line; other parts will be based on my personal experience.

One little bit of housekeeping: While Chapter 2, "Reflux 101," will help you understand the important difference between gastroesophageal reflux and gastroesophageal reflux disease, both are referred to as simply reflux, or acid reflux, at various points in the book. And you might assume from the title that *Colic Solved* is intended only for parents with babies in the first few months of life. While irritability is perhaps the most menacing symptom of reflux in babies, its symptoms can evolve over the first year of life. I intend, however, to carry you through the first year and into early toddlerhood, where the symptoms of reflux can linger.

You will find case histories and vignettes throughout the book. Remember that the standards of diagnosis and treatment vary considerably in different parts of the United States and among different doctors. They are presented only to illustrate the appearance of and potential approaches to particular problems. They are in no way intended to define a standard of therapy. The names have been changed to protect the innocent (cue *Dragnet* music), and any relationship to actual screaming babies is purely coincidental.

This book is not intended to replace or supersede anything that you may hear from your own gastroenterologist or pediatrician, should she be experienced and informed in the matters of spits, urps, and wet burps. There are a million ways to look at these problems and twice as many ways to approach them. Beyond the simplest form of the disease, you can't fix reflux yourself. You'll need to partner closely with your doctor. And no matter how little sleep you may get, your relationship with a great doctor will go far in advancing the happiness and well-being of your soon-to-be bundle of joy. This book should serve as a guide for you as you navigate the spotted and stained landscape of early childhood reflux. My greatest wish is for you to serve as an informed, empowered advocate for your screaming baby. Let this book be your guide. Let my voice be your narrator.

It's an exciting time to have a baby who screams and spits up everywhere—you're in the midst of a revolution! Be sure to check out colicsolved.com for new information, resources, and links. Complaints, concerns, and suggestions may be addressed to me personally at info@colicsolved.com. Happy reading, and stay dry.

COLIC SOLVED

1

THE TRUTH ABOUT
CRYING BABIES

I f your baby screams, she's not alone. It's estimated that about
1 of 5 babies have unexplained irritability. It's been 50 years
since the initial pigeonholing of irritable babies with a condition
that we've affectionately come to call colic. At the time that colic
was first described, doctors had few means of knowing what was
going on inside a baby. And in the absence of any better explanation, the idea of a five-letter word to sum it all up was warmly
received. And despite what we have come to know, colic as a
wastebasket diagnosis remains alive and well, a vestige of history
and a comfortable place to put the babies we have such a hard time
with. But your baby is screaming for a reason. It's a cry for help.

THE CASE OF BABY HANNAH

Hannah was 2 months old when she first visited me in my
Houston office. Her pediatrician had referred her because he
had exhausted all of his resources as a busy primary care pedi-

atrician. Hannah wouldn't stop crying, and he didn't know why. The best explanation this seasoned and reputable pediatrician had was that Hannah had colic.

Her problems began at around 2 weeks of age when she began crying after her feeding. Her crying progressed to throughout the day and started to affect her feeding. The pediatrician advised that her mother discontinue breastfeeding her because he feared that breast milk was the problem. Formula feeds began strong, but after a half ounce became difficult, with Hannah arching, pulling from the nipple, and in apparent pain, all while still being hungry and wanting more. The frustration of Hannah's hour-long feeding episodes were matched only by her sleep, which was regularly interrupted with piercing screams and painful gas.

Her waking hours were marked by nearly constant hiccups and the need to be held and moved. Hannah's parents were told that she had colic, yet colic medication never seemed to make much of a difference. Formula changes became nearly as frequent as diaper changes, but nothing seemed to make a difference.

The baby's incessant irritability, impossible feeding, and unpredictable sleeping patterns soon began to take its toll on her parents. When her mother returned to work when Hannah was 3 months old, understanding day care was hard to come by. At the end of their rope with a marriage at its limits, Hannah's parents came to see me.

WELCOME TO MY WORLD

Whether it's a pleasure or not, I have the opportunity to work with babies like Hannah every day. Thousands of screaming, miserable, sleepless, and impossible-to-feed babies have found their way to my office over the past several years, some sicker than others, but all delivered by desperate parents looking for answers and looking for help. This book is about what I've learned and what I know.

I've always said that it was far easier being a pediatrician before I ever had children of my own. Calls in the middle of the night from the sleepless parents of screaming babies were handled as a matter of course early on in my career. But despite my comforting words, my attitude beneath was "Deal with it." I had bought into the idea that all babies scream and that some babies scream because of the stress and pressure that young parents convey to their babies. While I have always done my best to evaluate and treat every baby thoroughly, I was very much inside the system at first . . . a paternalistic, board-certified know-it-all with 6 years of residency and fellowship training at America's largest children's hospital. But I had never lived with a baby. More important, I had never lived with a baby with reflux.

The birth of my daughter, Laura, represented a turning point for me as a pediatrician. Laura was a lot like Hannah, with the exception that her father was a pediatric gastroenterologist. And with that came expectations from my wife to make things better. Laura was treated for acid reflux and morphed from a bundle of misery to something far more tolerable. I was vindicated as both a father and a physician, and my view of the screaming baby has never been the same.

I should note that my son, Nicholas, happily spit everywhere and all the time until nearly a year of age. But for us this was nothing more than an inconvenience. In nearly all of his baby pictures, he is wearing a crusty burp bib intended to protect the expensive outfits we bought him as the firstborn. So you could say that I've had it both ways: a bundle of misery and a happy spitter, two patterns that you'll read about in Chapter 3, "Seven Signs of Reflux in Your Baby."

For better or worse, I can now empathize with the families I see—for better because I can understand their situation and react to it more sensitively; for worse because I can understand their situation and relive the misery that they feel whenever I'm called to evaluate a screamer.

COLIC—THE DIAGNOSIS FOR ALL OCCASIONS

Unfortunately, not everyone has a pediatric gastroenterologist as a father. In many cases, babies are left alone to cry, either by parents who don't know how to advocate for them or by doctors who don't know where to turn. In fact, in Hannah's case the diagnosis was colic because there was nothing else to explain her problem and the symptoms loosely fit with something that her pediatrician had been taught many years ago.

So What Is Colic?

The quest for the cause of colic or even an agreed-on definition of it over the last half century has amounted to something of an optical illusion. Like one of those abstract images that you must stare at for minutes on end before actually identifying the picture, colic has been something of an elusive diagnosis among pediatricians. And the many who never quite see it ultimately agree that they see it just so they won't have to continue squinting.

I'll have to admit that from early on in my career I was

never able to see the pretty picture when it came to the illusion of colic. While I've evaluated and treated thousands of irritable babies, the problem is that I've never seen colic and can't get straight answers about what it is or what it looks like from those who claim to have seen it. Like the UFOs that seem to land everywhere but at Harvard and MIT, colic has evolved into one of our culture's greatest urban legends—a mythical explanation meant to explain the seemingly unexplainable.

A Baby Cannot "Have" Colic

The problem comes with the fact that colic is a description and not a disease. This descriptive term has, in turn, been morphed into a real and recognizable condition that served an important role for parents and pediatricians in our not-so-distant past. Much as fables and myths help provide order and explanation for different cultures, colic was once a comfortable resting place for weary pediatricians dealing with weary parents. And when medical science failed to offer any better explanation, it served to conveniently absolve the pediatrician from any further responsibility to parent or child.

Because colic represents a pattern of behavior and not a disease, a baby cannot "have" colic or have it "diagnosed." Much like fever or weight loss that typically represents signs of some other problem in a child, colic doesn't stand on its own as a diagnosis. To use the words *diagnosis* and *colic* together suggests that intelligent, established criteria, backed up by clinical research, were used to come to that conclusion. But unfortunately, such criteria or compelling clinical studies don't exist. In the words of a distinguished researcher on the topic of infant irritability recently quoted in the *Journal of Pediatric Gastroen-*

terology and Nutrition, "The term colic implies a mechanism responsible for the distress displayed by these infants. Such a mechanism has never been demonstrated."

Colic—Whatever You Want It to Be

But colic advocates and researchers who have built their careers on the urban legend that is colic will beg to differ. The criterion they use, as determined in 1954, suggests that the diagnosis should be considered in babies who experience inconsolable screaming for 3 days a week, for 3 hours a day, for at least 3 weeks a month. Unfortunately, if your baby screams for only 2 hours and 45 minutes for only 20 days straight, you're a day early and a dollar short. Had I created criteria for colic, I would have suggested adding the fact that you haven't had sex with your spouse in 3 months, you're up 3 hours each night, and you're 3 weeks away from losing your job unless you get some sleep. But I wasn't practicing in the 1950s, and things were different then.

If we give our 1950s' researchers the benefit of the doubt and accept the out-of-thin-air rule of threes, as it is called, not everyone sticks to it. In fact, when it comes to the diagnosis of colic, everyone seems to have his or her own rules. A colleague whom I work closely with will diagnose colic only if the baby cannot be put down. Another employs a white-noise rule—the diagnosis is confirmed if the baby settles with the sound of a vacuum cleaner, hair dryer, or other loud neutralizing sound. It seems that the number of random, self-imposed criteria for diagnosis are limited only by the imagination.

So despite the complete absence of a consensus of what con-

BABY TYLER: THREE MONTHS CAME AND WENT

I first became suspicious when my pediatrician wanted to know the *exact* number of hours a day that Tyler spent screaming. As if I knew. I was having a hard enough time knowing what day it was, let alone keeping a scoresheet of his screaming. After just a few minutes in the exam room, "colic" was pronounced, as if the pediatrician was some kind of mind reader. "He'll be fine the day he hits three months," he said with a broad smile. "And trust me, someday you'll look back at this and laugh." He was gone about as quickly as he came. But 3 months came and went, and Tyler's misery never resolved. His feeding worsened, and he didn't gain weight as he was supposed to. Tyler was ultimately found to have reflux esophagitis by another doctor. Even to this day as I look back, amusement isn't the emotion that comes to mind.

stitutes colic, it remains nonetheless a convenient wastebasket diagnosis that can be retrofitted to suit the need of the individual making the diagnosis. If you haven't caught on, colic would appear to be a well-orchestrated five-letter defense mechanism for doctors who are either outdated, outwitted, or just plain out of ideas.

THE COLIC REVOLUTION—SCREAMING INTO THE TWENTY-FIRST CENTURY

Our experience and medical research tell us that babies scream for a reason. While *Colic Solved* doesn't intend to suggest that there aren't high-need babies or those with sensitive, developing nervous systems, it is here to introduce the idea that something physical may in fact be wrong.

In a sense, this book is the result of a revolution in pediatric medicine—a culmination of technology and insight. Advances in endoscopy (viewing the inside of body organs or cavities with a device that uses flexible fiber optics), pharmacology, and nutrition have allowed us to rethink why babies cry. In the twentieth century, we called it colic only because no one knew any better. And while developments in conquering diseases such as polio and smallpox obviously take center stage, other seemingly less impressive advances are important minor characters. Our understanding of the irritable baby is one of them.

Technology Has Changed Our Babies for the Better

So what are the changes in pediatric health care that have created a better understanding of why babies do what they do?

- *The creation of pediatric gastroenterology as a specialty.* While there have been pediatricians dedicated to the understanding of pediatric digestive health since the early 1900s, it was the formal organization of the field of pediatric gastroenterology that has created an atmosphere of organized discussion and research. The subspecialty of pediatric gastroenterology was recognized by the American Board of Medical Specialties in 1988, and since then the number of trained gastrointestinal (GI) specialists conducting research and setting the standards of care has continued to grow. Alongside the expansion of gastroenterology as a pediatric subspecialty has been the development of smaller endoscopes (flexible-tube optical instruments that use fiber optics to illuminate the inside of the intestinal tract) for understanding what happens in a baby's digestive system. pH probes came into popular use by pediatric gastroenterologists in the 1980s, allowing doctors to begin to associate patterns of reflux with patterns of irritability. (pH is a measure of acidity or alkalinity of a substance.)

- *Identification of reflux as a key contributor to a number of common conditions.* Beyond simply understanding acid reflux (the backflow of stomach acid into the esophagus, the muscular tube that carries food and drink to the stomach) in babies, this evolution of technology involving fiber-optic endoscopes and pH probes has allowed the correlation of reflux with other problems such as asthma, sinus conditions, and feeding disorders.
- *The advancement of infant nutrition.* Understanding of the growing immune system has led to the development of hypoallergenic formulas, specifically superhypoallergenic formula, which became available for common use in the early 1990s. This has revolutionized the care and feeding of the infant with severe allergic disease. Our ability to understand the reactions of the intestinal immune system has been furthered by our ability to "see" intestinal allergy with endoscopic technology. And while we continue to learn more and more about the incredible benefits of breastfeeding, formula manufacturers are learning from it to benefit babies who can't breastfeed. Formulas, which were once nothing more than a vehicle for protein, fat, and carbohydrate, now sometimes contain long-chain fatty acids that have been shown to improve visual and cognitive function in infancy and beyond.

- *The evolution of pediatric drug development.* The development and improvement of safe, effective antacids for use in children have revolutionized the way we see and care for the screaming baby. The technology of drug delivery has provided pediatricians with more options for facing the challenge of administering medicine to infants and children. And recent changes in federal law now mandate clinical trials (research studies) in children for many of the new drugs being released for adults.

- *The popularization of the Internet.* While many doctors consider it a curse, the Internet has empowered parents to network and ask questions about their baby's misery. Parents whose babies have been dealt the once dead-end diagnosis of colic now are learning in chat rooms and on Web sites that there may be identifiable and treatable problems at work. While the Web has the downside of sometimes offering too much information, its ability to raise questions is unparalleled.

So as we enter the twenty-first century, it sure seems like a great time to be a baby, particularly one who screams. All of these developments have made it easier to help the fussy baby.

Why Hannah Is Screaming

We now know that children with the type of irritability described as colic often suffer with either reflux or milk protein allergy.

A major study reported in 2004 by one of the world's most respected reflux researchers created quite a stir in the medical community. Clinical researchers treated a group of irritable babies with hypoallergenic formula. The babies whose symptoms didn't lessen when they were given hypoallergenic formula were then evaluated for the presence of gastroesophageal reflux using endoscopy and a pH probe (you'll learn more about these in Chapter 8, "A Parent's Guide to Tests and Studies," but for now understand that this is how reflux is formally assessed). Of 60 markedly irritable infants between the ages of 1 and 6 months, 66% had pH probe results consistent with abnormal reflux and 43% had evidence of acid reflux injury shown by biopsy of the esophagus. While the report's authors make it clear that proving an absolute cause-and-effect relationship between crying and obvious reflux can be difficult, the results are thought-provoking.

Even colic researchers are noting that there may be something more going on with the "colicky baby" than just a lot of crying. Another study reported in 2004 found a connection between infant colic and feeding difficulties. Forty-three percent of infants reported as having colic had what is referred to as disorganized feeding. And as we'll learn about in Chapter 3, "Seven Signs of Reflux in Your Baby," one of the most common causes of feeding difficulty in infancy is gastroesophageal reflux, or the passage of stomach contents up into the swallowing tube. So how many of the babies in this study had reflux? It's hard to say because none of the babies studied underwent a pH probe or endoscopy, which are the most common and reliable tools for diagnosing and quantifying reflux.

But as we'll learn, all that screams isn't reflux. In one of the most compelling studies looking at the relationship between colicky behavior and milk allergy, 27 infants with colic were treated with hypoallergenic formula, and a marked diminution in symptoms was seen in 24 of the infants. Coincidence? Well, the 24 infants were then given cow's milk formula in what's called a double-blind crossover study, meaning none of the observing parents knew whether their baby was being fed the second time with hypoallergenic formula or cow's milk formula. Of the 24 infants rechallenged with cow's milk protein, 18 showed a recurrence of their distress. So in this case, two thirds of the infants with "colic" showed dramatic and statistically significant improvement in their symptoms when treated with hypoallergenic formula.

Impressive statistics, but are these studies backed up with the experience of the real world? Yes, and that's what has inspired *Colic Solved*. I want to share with you what I've seen and what I've learned from the mothers and babies I have encountered in my practice. My experience, as well as that of many of my colleagues, is that the results reported are consistent with our own experiences. As I stated earlier in the chapter, while I have had thousands of babies referred for evaluation of unremitting colic, I have yet to diagnose or confirm "colic" in any of them.

So Do All Babies Who Cry Have Reflux?

Am I suggesting that every baby who cries has reflux or allergy? Of course not. Even the casual observer will see that not every baby in these studies had reflux or had symptoms that responded to treatment for allergy. And this is consistent with what we see in real life. There's a small percentage of miserable babies whose conditions physicians fail to diagnose or whose symptoms fail to respond to what we think they should respond to. And this is where the blob model comes in. One of the common misconceptions among new parents is that babies are creatures who do nothing more than eat, poop, sleep, and fuss. We like to think of them as all alike, angelic, cherublike blobs eating and sleeping until the day comes when their personality blossoms in a way that makes them different from every other baby in the neighborhood. But anyone who spends a lot of time with babies recognizes that despite the fact that they're all in the same receiving blankets, different babies have different temperaments, and each one is unique. Temperament influences how babies react to their environment. We can't change a baby's temperament; we can only work with it. In this way, babies are a lot like adults. They're all as different and unique as the adults we know.

So as it turns out, not all babies who cry have reflux. Differences in personality and temperament will influence how sensitive they are and how they react to the world around them.

You Can't Believe in Something You've Never Seen

Some doctors can't believe in something they've never seen. I have a friend who is a pharmaceutical salesperson in a rural Southern state selling a popular medication for endometriosis. As many women know, endometriosis is a fairly common condition that can lead to infertility and extremely painful periods. It's been the advancement in laparoscopic surgery within the past generation that has allowed gynecologists to recognize and treat endometriosis. But those physicians who haven't kept up to date and depend solely on their training from the early 1970s may overlook endometriosis. And so when my friend would make visits to inform physicians of her company's latest product for treating endometriosis, she would be met with empty stares and comments such as "We just don't see that much of

WHEN IT COMES TO BABIES MISERABLE WITH REFLUX, THE BREAST IS DEFINITELY BEST

It's interesting to note that colic gained popularity in the 1960s when the rates of breastfeeding were approaching an all-time low. While trying to draw a connection between rates of breastfeeding and the popularization of colic is practically impossible, we can say with certainty that breast milk is the best milk for babies suffering with reflux. As you'll learn in the pages ahead, infant reflux is in part a result of abnormal intestinal motility, or stomach squeezing. Breast milk is the easiest milk for babies to eliminate from the stomach and consequently one of the best foods to feed your miserable, refluxing baby.

it." They're right; they don't see that much of it because it isn't something that they think to look for. These are well-intentioned and otherwise experienced physicians who studied and trained in yesterday's world and for whom change doesn't come easy.

The endometriosis story is played out once again when it comes to pediatric reflux disease. Doctors years out of their training may not associate screaming in a baby or hoarseness in an older child with acid reflux disease. It's hard to identify something that you've never been taught to look for. I regularly speak on pediatric acid reflux, and I'm always amazed at the number of pediatricians who approach me after my presentation and comment, "I didn't know that some of these symptoms pointed to reflux. For years we've been calling this colic." And these aren't incompetents either. They're well-trained

practitioners who were never taught that inconsolable screaming, arching, and pulling from the nipple were symptoms of
anything other than colic. Like the babies suffering with this
condition and the parents who try to console them, they're vic-
tims as much as anyone else, trying to catch up with the advances in medicine that are now giving us explanations and
answers.

IF YOU DON'T CARE, MAYBE NO ONE ELSE WILL

Too small to ask for help, your baby can communicate only
through her cries and patterns of behavior. It's up to you to
serve as her advocate and try to change her situation by recognizing the obvious signs of a very treatable condition. If your
pediatrician has made it a habit to diagnose every fussy baby's
condition as colic, you need to be suspicious and ask informed
questions. You should make it clear that you want all treatable
conditions ruled out.

You'll need to trust your instincts. When baby Hannah was
in my office, the visit was interrupted by a call from the referring doctor to fill me in on some of the details of her case. I was
warned that there was "probably nothing wrong with the
baby" and that the parents were having a hard time coping
with this, their first baby. So when all else fails, some physicians imply that the parents are crazy. In the end, Hannah was
successfully treated for reflux esophagitis and, within 2 to 3
weeks of starting therapy, she was feeding and sleeping without a hitch.

My mother liked to say that worrying would never accom-
plish anything, but concern is what drives you to keep your
children safe and well. Fear is the fuel that keeps parents on

cue and children out of danger. I can't count the number of times that I have gone the extra yard on being pushed by the intuition of a concerned parent, only to be proven wrong. So I've learned to follow the philosophy of the guys from *Ghost Busters*, whose motto was "We're ready to believe you."

SCREAMING AT THE BABY WHISPERER

Our culture perpetuates the belief that the screaming baby is a parenting problem. Bookstores are filled with manuals and guides that perpetuate the concept that there's really never anything wrong with the baby and that all you need to do is whisper in just the right way and make the proper shushing noise. It always seems to be that parents are failing to read cues and act in the way that good parents are supposed to act. We're overrun with nineteenth-century nanny wisdom that has parents everywhere feeling incompetent.

THE ANATOMY OF THE FOURTH TRIMESTER

Harvey Karp, M.D., author of the best-selling *Happiest Baby on the Block*, may have been onto something when he began popularizing the concept of a fourth trimester, in which the baby brain isn't quite ready to be out in the world. The same may be true for the gut. If we buy into the argument that there really is a fourth trimester and it's the failure to adapt to this that leads babies to scream inconsolably, we have to look at the functioning of the intestinal tract during this period. As you'll see in Chapter 2, "Reflux 101," there are specific issues with the intestinal tract that are common in the most irritable babies with spitting. Motility, or squeezing, of the intestinal tract is often delayed in

"OF COURSE I'M CRAZY—MY BABY SCREAMS FOURTEEN HOURS A DAY"

Parents are often the ones held accountable when their babies scream. Physicians can use terms such as *parental stress* and *poor adjustment* to defer responsibility away from themselves and onto parents. After all, if you were a good parent, you would know how to make your baby happy, right? Wrong. While it is important to understand that different babies have different temperaments, painful screaming typically occurs for a reason. Recognize and believe that you are not to blame. Your efforts in asking questions are a testimony to your love for your baby.

babies. This delay usually is due to the immaturity of the intestinal system and improves with time (remarkably, just like colic), but it also can arise from intestinal inflammation caused by milk protein allergy. Alas, the intolerable screaming of some newborns may be a consequence not of the parents' not knowing how to cope with the fourth trimester or not picking the appropriate shushing noise but rather of the parents' failure to advocate for their children by asking the appropriate questions and seeking appropriate care. Actually, calming techniques are important even for babies irritable from reflux or allergy. But while the nanny-granny wisdom espoused by *Secrets of the Baby Whisperer* and *The Happiest Baby on the Block* may have its role for the baby with the fidgets, its application to the exclusion of seeking medical care in the seriously irritable baby can lead to the oversight of easily treatable conditions.

Unfortunately, the evaluation and treatment of the screaming baby isn't always straightforward. Parents are different, babies are different, and the way they show their problems can vary tremendously. Getting the best care for your child requires vigilance. Let this book serve as a starting point for understanding that the answer to your baby's pain lies not in a rigid schedule, a shushing sound, or a wrapping technique but rather in the belief that your baby's pain is treatable and real.

A WORD ABOUT COLIC, QUACKS, AND PROFESSIONAL RISK

One of my colleagues has suggested that my views on colic should probably be kept close to my chest. A veteran of nearly 30 years and doctor to thousands of babies in south Texas, he's let me know in no uncertain terms that undermining one of the twentieth century's greatest safe havens for pediatricians could be harmful to my professional health. But my opinions are already well known in my community, and for years I have been telling families that I'm still looking for my first case of colic. Why stop now?

The fact is that infant reflux should be on every responsible pediatrician's radar. NASPGHAN recently undertook a national education campaign on this matter. The literature is flush with information that supports the fact that many of these miserable babies have a treatable condition. Word is out.

My views represent a mix of clinical science, intuition, and experience brought together for you, the reader. I'm fortunate to have worked since 1991 at Texas Children's Hospital in Houston's Texas Medical Center, where there is a vibrant, educated pediatric medical community that stays abreast of the latest advances. Much of what I've learned about reflux disease

HOW THIS BOOK WILL HELP YOU TO HELP YOUR BABY—THREE STEPS

1. *Be vigilant.* If you have a "colicky" baby, this book will give you the tools you need to be able to recognize the symptoms of reflux.
2. *Advocate for your child.* Knowing about infant reflux will allow you to advocate for your baby.
3. *Get the proper help.* The system may be stacked against you. By knowing what questions to ask and what to expect, you can get your baby the help she needs.

has come from them, the physicians who have referred so many patients. Together we've sorted out a lot of these issues and worked to bring them to the forefront. I'm also fortunate to have trained with some of pediatric gastroenterology's early pioneers. And the greatest influence, of course, has been those hundreds if not thousands of parents who brought their screaming babies branded with the great big *C* on their foreheads. It has been their stories as well as the successes and failures of working with their babies that has taught me the most.

2

REFLUX 101

So maybe there's a chance that your baby's painful screaming is the result of a treatable condition. Perhaps your baby has gastroesophageal reflux. What is reflux, and how did your baby get it?

DEFINING REFLUX—"WHAT GOES DOWN MIGHT COME UP"

Very simply, gastroesophageal reflux (GER) describes the physiologic condition in which stomach contents come back up from the stomach into the esophagus where it doesn't belong. Notice that this definition says nothing about having symptoms or being sick. Reflux doesn't necessarily have to give a baby symptoms. In fact, reflux is a *physiologic* process, which means that it's normal. In fact, it may surprise you to learn that all babies have reflux. Day in and day out, your child and the baby next door experience reflux. Up and down, up and down, hour in and

BABY KYLLIE: SCREAMING, SCREAMING EVERYWHERE BUT NEVER ONCE A SPIT-UP

Kyllie was almost 4 months old before our pediatrician diagnosed reflux. She screamed and arched, and formula changes didn't seem to help. Because Kyllie never vomited or spit up, we never thought reflux could be possible. And because her symptoms were worse in the evening, we thought it was colic. At her 4-month checkup when we discussed her symptoms further with the pediatrician, we learned that babies can get reflux esophagitis without ever spitting up.

hour out, and you may not even know it—because in an otherwise healthy baby, it doesn't present a problem in most cases. It is a normal process that occurs in everyone. It's called *physiologic reflux*.

Sometimes this passage of stomach contents up into the esophagus isn't so innocent, however. The acid that makes up refluxed material can irritate the esophagus and upper airway such that symptoms develop. When these symptoms interfere with a baby's day-to-day activity, reflux is referred to as gastroesophageal reflux disease (GERD), or *pathologic reflux*. This is physiologic reflux gone bad.

This difference between GER and GERD is key. It helps us discriminate reflux as a laundry problem from reflux as a medical problem. Babies with GER are those who spit but don't suffer any consequences. This is your average happy, healthy, growing baby with wet burps. Babies with GERD, on the other hand, typically have problems relating to feeding, growth, or breathing as a consequence of their reflux. We identify them as sick babies who need medical attention. So while all babies have some degree of GER, fewer suffer from GERD. We'll discuss the symptoms and patterns of GERD in much more detail in the next chapter.

WHY IS REFLUX SUCH A COMMON PROBLEM FOR INFANTS?

Everyone, including you the reader and your baby, has reflux throughout the day. But despite this seemingly universal human experience, we never see adults walking around with burp cloths. Babies' reflux seems to be special. It may not be that it's more common in babies but rather that there are elements of infant physiology and anatomy in the upper intestinal tract that make reflux more apparent and lead to reflux symptoms. See the Appendix for illustrations of a baby's upper intestinal anatomy.

"The Faulty Valve"

At the bottom of the esophagus (swallowing tube), right before it enters the stomach, there is a circular ring of muscles called the *lower esophageal sphincter* (LES) that helps keep stomach contents where they belong. The LES works pretty hard to stay closed, but in babies it can't squeeze as strong as it can in an adult, and it undergoes frequent episodes of relaxation. When this occurs, stomach contents are allowed to flow back into the esophagus. These transient relaxations become few and far between as a baby gets older and the LES grows into its job. By the time babies are 3 to 6 weeks old, the LES pressure reaches that of adults.

If you talk to enough parents of reflux babies, most per-
ceive their child's problem as an issue with this sphincter, or
"valve." (While I try to avoid referring to the LES as a valve,
years of hearing the usage from parents has got me saying it
myself.) Often the first question that comes up is "Can the
valve be fixed?" The short answer is no, although you will read
about an operation in Chapter 7 ("Medications for Reflux: To
Treat or Not to Treat?") that's used in sick babies to control reflux when medicines can't. And as we'll see, reflux in infants
goes well beyond 1 or 2 months of age, which tells us that reflux is more than just an LES issue.

While the inconvenience of LES relaxations in babies may
create wet burps, it's likely nature's way of keeping your baby
happy. Babies naturally swallow air during the course of feeding, and without some natural means of allowing this air to decompress, they would be remarkably uncomfortable.

Poor Stomach Emptying

It should be obvious from the descriptions so far that reflux is a
problem in which a baby's stomach contents move in the wrong
direction. Physicians characterize this type of problem as a
motility disorder. Motility disorders can affect any part of the
intestines. Constipation, for example, can result from poor
motility, or squeezing, of the lower intestinal tract.

One of the major factors contributing to reflux in infants is
delayed emptying of the stomach. We've learned that the
stomach undergoes regular squeezing that facilitates digestion
and helps food leave the stomach. Under normal circumstances
a liquid meal, for example, should be gone from a baby's stomach in approximately 30 to 60 minutes. During the first several

months of a baby's life, the stomach is inefficient at emptying, and milk has a tendency to sit around longer than it should. Consequently, it's not uncommon for a baby to spit up 2 to 3 hours after a feed. While this isn't considered normal, it's common enough that physicians consider this nothing more than a delay in intestinal development.

Slower Intestinal Motility

When a physician puts pressure balloons into the intestinal tract of a baby and measures the patterns of squeezing, he sees a very different pattern from that of an adult. Under normal circumstances, in adults there are waves of squeezing, commonly referred to as *migrating motor complexes* (MMCs). These MMCs are responsible for propelling food and nutrients through the intestinal tract. MMCs are present in babies but move at half the speed and half the strength of those in adults. While these findings don't directly contribute to reflux in newborns, it should be quite apparent that things aren't moving as quickly or efficiently in babies.

Positioning

Young infants spend the majority of their time in the horizontal position. It isn't too hard to understand that when a baby lies flat, it's easier for stomach contents to flow into the esophagus. In adults, gravity normally helps to keep reflux in check. Until your baby begins to sit up (at about age 6 months), you can expect gravity to contribute to the problem.

While we're on the subject of positioning, I should mention something about belly versus back positioning. As a rule, babies with reflux tend to do better on their stomachs. This is because the LES lies closer to a baby's back. When they are positioned on their stomachs, milk tends to settle forward, thereby avoiding the LES. When babies lie on their backs, milk tends to pool near the LES, waiting for that next relaxation and the opportunity to come up and out. But as most parents know, how we position a baby for sleep may be related to sudden infant death syndrome (SIDS). So we'll talk about positioning for sleep in more detail in Chapter 6, "The Care and Handling of Your Crying, Spitting, Difficult-to-Soothe Baby."

Relative to their size, babies are subjected to significant changes in posture and position that make regurgitation all the more likely. While it's hard to believe that all that huggin' and sugar could somehow be bad for your little spitter, it only makes sense. Think of how your reflux would be if, after a surf-and-turf dinner, you were put on your back to have your bottom wiped with a cold, wet towel, then picked up by your midsection, and then held over your captor's head, only to be tickled unmercifully. When it comes to reflux, gravity never lies.

Not-So-Efficient Feeding

The way your baby feeds can influence her reflux. One of the unfortunate consequences of being an inexperienced feeder is not-so-efficient feeding. Whenever your baby latches and creates a seal on the bottle or breast, a little bit of air gets swallowed. Additional air in the stomach creates distention and the need to burp, both of which are a setup for acid reflux. Once your baby has plenty of practice, this contributor to reflux will disappear.

Liquid Diet

When you consider poor stomach emptying, a weak LES valve, and nearly round-the-clock horizontal positioning, an all-liquid diet can only make matters worse. Unlike expensive ketchup that's hard to shake out of a bottle, liquid refluxes easier than solids. And it's probably no coincidence that reflux becomes less common as solids become a larger part of a baby's diet late in the first year.

WHY REFLUX MAY BE A BIGGER PROBLEM FOR OUR BABIES THAN IT IS FOR US

Pediatricians Tend to Overlook It

Reflux is potentially more dangerous in babies and children because as family physicians and pediatricians, we are inclined to think that it doesn't exist and that when it does exist, it isn't a problem. My favorite one-liner from referring pediatricians is "Reflux is a laundry problem, not a medical problem." This unfortunate and outdated attitude ignores a very real problem and puts some babies at risk.

Reflux in infancy and childhood is more frequently overlooked than in adulthood because physicians who treat adults are trained to look for it. Adults are inundated with direct-to-consumer advertising warning them of the subtle symptoms that they need to look for. Children are different. While it has been estimated that 7 million children younger than age 17 have symptomatic reflux, I have been faced by seasoned pediatricians who say that they have yet to see a case of any significance in their career. Scary but true. Ignorance is bliss, and it's hard to believe in something that you think you've never seen. So our children are in a tougher position with reflux than adults are because it may be difficult to get their symptoms taken seriously. But it's encouraging that pediatric reflux is gaining respect as a real medical condition deserving of attention.

Babies Can't Talk; They Can Only Scream

It's been said that the job of pediatrician is a lot like that of veterinarian—the patients can't talk. This can create problems if we don't pay attention to the warning signs of reflux disease in our babies. Unlike adults, who can watch TV, read, and go see a physician, our babies depend on us to advocate for them. And if we listen closely enough and keep an open mind, we'll often hear the signs of reflux in our screaming, miserable babies.

Reflux Is a Great Imitator

Beyond the fact that babies can't talk to us, the reflux picture is complicated further by the fact that it can look like so many other things:

- *Something in the air tonight:* In Houston, where getting rid of mold infestation in homes has become something of an industry, parents often try to tie their baby's congestion to environmental spores. But we know that infants with chronic reflux will often suffer with noisy breathing and congestion much like that in an individual with environmental allergies.
- *Lonely or in pain?* Nighttime awakening, a common behavioral problem during late infancy and early toddler-

hood, can sometimes be the only symptom of burning nocturnal reflux esophagitis.

- *"It's obviously the parent."* Reflux may masquerade as poor parenting. Reflux symptoms are commonly blamed on parents, who are told that they're overfeeding, feeding too frequently, transferring stress, or spoiling their baby. But very often the parent is responding to a dreadfully unhappy, hungry infant who is losing calories to reflux and is in pain.

- *Nipples and things:* The feeding problems commonly seen in the refluxing infant are often attributed to use of the wrong bottle system. But as we will learn, the feeding difficulties of the baby with esophagitis have little to do with pricey bottle systems, nipples, or flow rates.

Earlier Reflux Can Mean Earlier Complications

Sometimes the most severe cases of reflux, certainly those involving toddlers, can add up to earlier complications. Scarring of the esophagus, chronic lung disease, and feeding disorders can result from poorly managed reflux in babies and toddlers. While this is the exception, we must be vigilant of what our babies are telling us when they scream, choke, and can't feed.

THE HIDDEN EPIDEMIC?

It's hard to say exactly how common reflux disease is in babies. The difficulty in coming up with statistics lies in the fact that reflux symptoms can range from mild to dramatic, with all shades of gray in between. Numerous disorders can have signs

REFLUX BY THE NUMBERS

- Close to 70% of babies between 4 and 6 months old spit up at least once a day.
- About 5% of 1-year-olds spit up at least once a day at their first birthday.
- Babies with frequent spitting are 2.3 times more likely than infrequent spitters to have reflux at age 9 years.
- About 8% of all teenagers report regular reflux symptoms.

and symptoms similar to those of reflux, making precise analysis difficult. But if we look at spitting up as the most frequently recognized sign of reflux, studies show that 67% of 4-month-old infants have GER. This number drops to 5% in 1-year-olds. It has been estimated that 1 in 10 older children are symptomatic with their GER. Some experts who treat reflux believe that these numbers fall short of the true incidence of the disease. The bottom line is that if your child has symptoms of reflux, you're definitely not alone.

Described by some as the hidden epidemic, reflux certainly has become a common diagnosis for babies in recent years. The question is: Is there actually more reflux these days, or are we identifying it more readily now? My guess is that it's the latter, although there are no good studies looking at reflux diagnosis in the past versus now to prove what's really going on. When you talk to the old-time pediatricians and describe a fussily feeding baby with frequent spitting, he or she would most likely describe that as a normal condition of infancy—and for good reason. Reflux truly is a normal condition of infancy and comes under the disease category only when a baby can't feed, grow, or breathe properly.

As the tricks and tools for diagnosing and treating the subtle variants of reflux have improved, so has physicians' interest in looking for it. Parents read or hear about it and want to know if their child has it. Pediatricians sometimes enjoy the satisfaction of labeling a condition for tired, concerned parents who want answers. Pediatric gastroenterology has evolved so that we have small endoscopes for investigating the complications of reflux and pH meters for coming up with a diagnosis in the trickiest cases. The nutrition and pharmaceutical industry has gotten into the mix with new formulas and wonder drugs. We've created a cottage industry of sorts that seems to perpetuate itself. More than likely, reflux is no more common now than it was in the 1970s. It's just that we have new ways to look at an old problem.

REFLUX GENETICS

Possibly the question I get asked most frequently from young parents of babies with severe reflux is "If I have more children, will they have reflux too?" And they ask for good reason. When your life has been turned upside down by a baby with severe reflux, you want to do everything you can to avoid a repeat performance.

Some of the common issues in babies that can lead to acid reflux include extra relaxation of the LES, poor stomach emptying, and even excessive acid production, so we know that reflux in babies is more than just one problem attributable to one genetic defect. Consequently, the combination of physiologic

DON'T LET A SOUR APPLE SPOIL THE BUNCH

It's been said that "colicky" behavior from reflux esophagitis is the best birth control. I can't count the number of young parents who have reported to me that they are not interested in having more children over fear of having another with severe reflux. While I can appreciate the mind-numbing effect of sleep deprivation and incessant marital discord, keep in mind that all of this will pass. Acid reflux in babies is typically a time-limited problem. While reflux disease does have genetic roots, your experience with reflux in one baby doesn't necessarily seal your fate as far as your next child is concerned. Most parents who experience reflux esophagitis with one baby don't see it with subsequent children.

problems that may have made your first child so miserable are unlikely to appear together in subsequent children.

With that said, however, there are some issues regarding the genetics of reflux that are worth talking about. Experience with thousands of such children teaches that there are heritable conditions that can lead some children to have reflux that is more severe than that of the average bear. Let's talk about a few examples of reflux genetics in action:

Hiatal Hernia

Remember that the esophagus passes down in the chest, through the diaphragm, and into the abdomen, where it empties into the stomach. The LES that holds stomach contents where they belong sits about at the level of the diaphragm. In some families, the opening in the diaphragm that allows the esophagus to pass through is unusually large. When this is the case, a situation exists where organs that normally stay put in the abdominal cavity can slide up into the chest where they don't belong. This is referred to as a hiatal hernia.

In children with hiatal hernia, the stomach can slide up into the chest through this diaphragm defect. Now, under normal circumstances, having a small piece of the stomach slip into the chest on occasion isn't a crime. In fact, most children grow quietly into adulthood without any problems. People with hiatal hernia lack the support offered by the diaphragm in holding stomach contents in the stomach. And as you can imagine, the sliding of stomach in and out of this opening makes it easier for acid to slip up into the esophagus.

So what does any of this have to do with genetics? As it turns out, hiatal hernias love company; when Mom, Dad, or a grandparent has a hiatal hernia, the odds of a child in the family developing one is significant. And for children with hiatal hernia, reflux tends to be a bit more difficult to treat. In fact, in older children with hiatal hernia whose symptomatic reflux fails to respond to medical therapy, surgical repair can be the best option.

Barrett's Esophagus

Barrett's esophagus is a precancerous change that occurs in the lining of the esophagus in people with severe reflux. Typically, this is a condition of adulthood, although it occasionally occurs in children with long-standing, severe reflux disease. Most commonly, a child with Barrett's esophagus has a parent with either Barrett's esophagus or severe reflux. While there are

THE REFLUX GENE—COULD MY CHILD HAVE IT?

With all the research on the human genome, it seems today that there's a gene for everything, and reflux seems to be no exception. A large group of families with children with severe reflux were recently studied, and all were found to have an abnormality of a gene on chromosome 13. Genes represent sequences of DNA (deoxyribonucleic acid) that code for certain products that our body produces. As it turns out, the gene that these researchers identified as abnormal in these families codes for a special nerve transmitter in the intestinal tract. And as we already know, one of the problems behind GER in children is abnormal squeezing of the intestinal tract. But don't run to a geneticist just yet. It is thought that a number of physiologic problems come together to create the symptoms seen in children with reflux. This genetic defect, though fascinating, probably represents the root of reflux in only a small fraction of patients.

other genetic factors that can influence cells to become precancerous, the familial role of severe reflux is known to be a factor. Barrett's esophagus is unheard of in infants, but its occasional presence in young children with severe reflux supports some role of genetics in reflux.

Double Reflux

When I think about genetics and reflux, I recall a family that I cared for early in my practice. The parents had had difficulty conceiving and resorted to in vitro fertilization. As is often the case with assisted fertility, the mother carried multiple ba-

HE CRIED, SHE CRIED

Studies suggest that there are slightly more boys than girls who have GERD in infancy. This discrepancy between the sexes holds true in adulthood. The reason for this difference in infancy isn't known, but in adults, it could be due to genetic and hormonal factors.

bies—four beautiful babies. Though healthy at birth, the babies shortly began to experience symptoms of spitting, difficulty feeding, and profound irritability. I should emphasize that *all four* babies had these symptoms when I was called on to help them. The first time in my office was a sight to behold, with two tandem strollers and two nannies in tow, the babies screaming, and the parents distraught not only from lack of sleep but also from having to bring the children clear across town and into the Texas Medical Center.

It was impressive that all the babies had similar patterns of regurgitation, feeding, and pain, suggesting that there was some heritable factor that all the babies acquired that made them so miserable with reflux. And interestingly, all four babies' symptoms resolved at about the same time late in the first year. My observations were not unfounded. Studies have shown that among twins, identical twins are more likely than nonidentical twins to share reflux symptoms. So whatever a baby's mechanism of reflux, be it poor squeezing of the stomach or overproduction of acid, it appears that it may be replicated in children who share the same genes.

After this family's valiant effort to bring their children to my office, I offered to make house calls thereafter (one of the few times in my career). And the experience was one that I won't forget. The scene at home was only slightly less chaotic than that observed in my office. The house, an obviously beautiful home in its day, was now overturned and retrofitted for nannies, live-in loved ones, and four newborns. Beyond the obvious chaos that one would expect, what I recall most clearly was the continuous screaming and the piles of burp cloths on every armrest and table. While these babies had some improvement with treatment, the level of care that they required took its toll on the desperate parents, who, sadly, were divorced within 2 years. Beyond the genetics of reflux, this case demonstrates the impact of esophagitis and multiple births on a marriage.

3

SEVEN SIGNS OF REFLUX
IN YOUR BABY

So how do you know if your baby's screaming and "colicky" symptoms are caused by reflux? Actually, all babies have reflux to some degree. On the one end of the reflux spectrum are the babies with normal physiologic reflux who do nothing more than spit up a little bit. Parents may gripe about it, but it's usually nothing more than an inconvenience. At the other end of the spectrum are babies who are sick with reflux. These are the babies with screaming, arching, difficulty feeding, and even poor growth and breathing problems. Both the healthy babies and the sick babies are typically easy to pick out. It's the babies whose symptoms lie between the two extremes who can be challenging. Knowing when a baby has crossed that line into needing treatment or special care requires a great deal of experience and understanding of babies with this problem. It's important to know that even physicians argue about how much is too much when it comes to the symptoms of baby heartburn.

THE SEVEN SIGNS OF REFLUX IN INFANCY

While it would be easy to generate a laundry list of every little thing a refluxing baby can do, let's stick with seven of the most common signs and symptoms that parents see when their baby is suffering with reflux.

1. Spitting and Vomiting

Spits, Urps, and Wet Burps
The telltale sign of reflux in a baby is the presence of the spit-up or wet burp. But all babies spit up at some point, don't they? They sure do, and that's how we can so confidently say that all babies have reflux. In fact, 70% of all 4-month-old babies spit up at least once a day.

The technical term for spitting up is *regurgitation*, and it represents the passive flow of stomach contents up through the esophagus and out of the mouth. Regurgitation occurs when the valve above the stomach relaxes at the same time that pressure is produced around the stomach (such as during cuddling, handling, or position changes). Milk takes the path of least resistance, and up it comes. And when you consider that babies frequently have slow tummy emptying, the backflow of milk becomes easier to understand.

Some parents are concerned by the appearance of spit-up and the way that babies spit up:

- *Spit-up that looks like clabbered milk:* You may notice a white, cheesy material present on your baby's burp cloth. It should be no cause for concern. When the protein found in milk is exposed to the strong acid found in a baby's

THE SEVEN SIGNS

The presence of one or more of the following signs may suggest that your baby is suffering with GERD:

1. Spitting and vomiting
2. Constant hiccups
3. Feeding disturbances
4. Chronic irritability
5. Discomfort when lying on the back
6. Sleep disturbance
7. Chronic cough and/or congestion

stomach, it undergoes a normal curdling reaction. All babies convert milk protein to this lumpy, acrid-smelling substance, but fortunately it usually stays in the stomach, never to be seen. The presence or absence of this curdled milk protein in your child's spit-up has no relationship to the severity of his reflux.

- *Spit-up that comes out of the nose:* Parents are universally worried when their child spits or vomits through the nose. If you have the pleasure of witnessing this lovely variant of normal reflux, it shouldn't cause concern. This most likely represents a mild difference in your child's anatomy that facilitates material taking a detour back through the sinuses rather than straight out of the mouth. Time and growth are often helpful in straightening things out.
- *Spit-up that contains mucus:* If cheesy curds aren't enough to upset you, mucus may be. But not to worry. The stomach

is one of the many organs in our body that creates mucus to help lubricate and move intestinal contents along. Mucus can also come from sinus drainage. Babies suffering with upper respiratory infections very often have a lot of mucus in their spit-up. In either case, the presence of mucus on a baby's burp cloth is no reason for heartburn of your own.

- *Spitting up that happens 2 hours after eating:* You may notice that your baby spits up right to the minute before her next feed. This is concerning to most new parents because it appears as though the regurgitation is constant and it creates the perception that digestion isn't taking place. This delay is typically nothing to worry about and represents what we already know about babies: Their tummies empty slowly. While not necessarily normal, it is very common among babies with reflux.

Vomiting

As parents and even pediatricians, we unfortunately have a tendency to throw around terms such as *spitting* and *vomiting*. But there is a difference between the two terms. And it's useful to try to be precise in describing what's going on with our children because how food comes out sometimes gives us information as to why it's coming out. In contrast to spitting up, vomiting is a forceful, sometimes violent process in which the stomach is cleared of its contents. From a physiologic perspective, it is very coordinated and involves powerful wringing of the stomach, relaxation of the valve at the bottom of the esophagus, closure of the airway, and tearing of the eyes. While most babies with reflux will typically regurgitate, sometimes they will start out with a small retch, or urp, which causes them to gag and vomit.

So what does it mean if your baby just vomits? By itself, vomiting doesn't have to mean anything serious. What is important are the other symptoms that may accompany it.

- *Is the baby able to feed and gain weight?* This is often the ultimate bottom line when it comes to establishing a baby's wellness.
- *What is the quality of the vomiting?* Is it forceful, or is there yellow bile material that might suggest an upper intestinal obstruction?
- *Are there physical findings to suggest that the baby is sick?* Distention of the abdomen, significant pain, poor skin color, low muscle tone, or a heart murmur might be a clue that your baby's vomiting is a sign of something more sinister.

While you should always be vigilant of the symptoms noted above, only your physician can determine which physical findings represent a problem and which are just a speed bump in your baby's development.

Rumination—The Wet Burp That Never Quite Got There

It's important to add that infants don't necessarily have to regurgitate or vomit to have reflux. Some of the sickest babies I have ever treated never spit up a day in their short lives. Stomach contents can pass from the stomach up into the upper esophagus, creating irritation along the way and yet never creating so much as a wet burp. Parents will often describe the sound of "food coming up," which can be associated with "colicky" behavior, irritability, lip-smacking, and swallowing. These symptoms are sometimes referred to as *rumination*, and unless a physician has

REFLUX RASH

Parents frequently struggle with chin and neck irritation in their spitting baby. In most cases the irritation comes from the acid and pepsin found in stomach contents, but look out for the presence of a red, prickly rash with cheesy white material in the neck of the chubbier baby. It can look like clabbered milk, but it may be a yeast infection, given the constant exposure to moisture. Remember:

- Keep the chin and neck clean and dry.
- Consider small amounts of creams such as Aquaphor or zinc oxide to keep moisture out.
- Consult your physician about any persistent rash with cheesy white material. This could represent a yeast infection.

taken a careful history, this subtle symptom of reflux may go overlooked. Rumination is a wet burp that never quite got there.

2. Constant Hiccups

Hiccups represent spasm or twitching of the diaphragm (the large muscle that separates the chest from the abdomen). The diaphragm normally contracts regularly to allow us to take in even, slow breaths. When the diaphragm contracts or twitches suddenly, a small amount of air is taken in. As this occurs, the vocal cords immediately snap shut, causing the sound that we typically associate with a hiccup. This closing of the vocal cords probably represents an effort by the body to prevent the inhalation of food during the hiccup.

HOW CAN THEY GAIN WEIGHT WITH
ALL THAT SPITTING UP?

I'm frequently confronted by concerned grandmothers who tell me that "this amount of spitting is not normal," after which I hear with absolute insistence that "there's no way that this baby could be growing with all the formula she's losing." Concern over growth in the baby who frequently spits up is common. But just like picky toddlers who have a knack for taking in what they need to grow, most babies have a remarkable capacity to compensate for lost calories. This is typically made up through feeding more frequently or more aggressively. This natural ability to adjust for caloric loss is one of the reasons that I typically do not recommend restriction of volumes or "scheduling" in the refluxing baby. Feeding babies less may result in smaller urps, but they will remain hungry, frustrated, and irritable, all sensations that will increase crying, air swallowing, and ultimately reflux.

Despite the fact that all babies experience hiccups from time to time, babies with reflux experience hiccups more often. When I ask parents about the presence of frequent hiccups, I'm often met with a look of surprise as if I've somehow read their minds. All along, they've wondered if their baby's hiccups actually meant something. The hiccups these parents describe are frequent and sometimes painful to watch. While it has never been reported in the medical literature, the mothers of some of the sickest babies with reflux whom I see have reported that their babies experienced nearly constant hiccups in utero. Remember that reflux is a motility disturbance and the intestines are quite active long before a baby is born.

There aren't any quick-and-dirty solutions for hiccups in your baby. For the infant with reflux, treatment may be all that's necessary. Otherwise, the only good option is to distract or comfort your baby until the hiccups go away.

3. Feeding Disturbances

Poor Feeding

No discussion of reflux or esophagitis would be complete without looking at its impact on feeding. As you may be able to imagine, an irritated throat and esophagus make for painful swallowing. When babies hurt, they're typically not interested in eating. This creates a real dilemma for infants, because when they're hungry, they want to eat. What you will likely observe in babies with reflux esophagitis is a very disorganized, chaotic feeding pattern. The desire to eat will lead to an intense interest in the nipple, which, after a few sucks, results in a grimace and pulling away from the breast or bottle. Once away, the baby realizes how hungry she really is and tries again. This cycle repeats itself over and over again for 30 to 60 minutes until either the child or the parent becomes so exhausted that they finally give up.

Because of the child's impaired intake, the parents feel compelled to try feeding the baby sooner than her normal schedule would dictate. And as the baby is hungry from getting only half her normal volume during the last feed, she's also ready earlier. But then the same feeding pattern repeats itself. Feeding ultimately becomes a dreaded exercise for parents

BABY EMMA: "WE THOUGHT IT WAS JUST GAS"

It seemed that Emma's gas was the cause of her nonstop screaming. The gas was painful and she was loud. We tried all of the over-the-counter remedies, but they didn't seem to make a difference. Everyone said that this type of gas is common with colic, so we just lived with it. When we switched pediatricians, we learned that Emma's gas was actually caused by air that she was swallowing during her hour-long feeding marathons. No one had ever asked us how long it was taking our baby to feed. When we finally treated her reflux, her feeding became more efficient and organized and her gas went away.

who, day in and day out, spend hours desperately trying to nourish their baby.

One interesting pattern that parents may notice is an improvement in feeding at nighttime. When babies with severe reflux esophagitis are half asleep, they'll often feed much better. In fact, some parents will report that the majority of their child's meager daily intake comes in the middle of the night. Why is this? More than likely, the sleeping baby isn't quite as aware of the pain that usually keeps her from feeding well. When babies are relaxed, the coordination of sucking and swallowing happens more easily.

Voracious Feeding
As strange as it may sound, the exact opposite feeding pattern can also be seen with esophagitis. Some babies will feed fast and furious like there's no tomorrow. While it may have been only 2½

hours since their last feed, they'll behave as if they haven't fed in hours. Sucking and swallowing may seem aggressive and even desperate. In their desperation for more milk faster, they will frequently squeak and slurp. These babies are feeding for the relief that feeding brings. For whatever reason, the combination of physiologic factors (remember that reflux is the end result of a handful of problems that can occur in any combination) that have led to these babies' reflux are soothed by the flow of milk.

Gas, an Unexpected Consequence of Feeding Problems

My son's great-grandmother suggested that his gas was the result of spending too much time outside on windy days. For normal babies, there may be something to this, but for the baby with reflux, there is a better explanation.

Babies with reflux are typically quite gassy. In fact, parents will often assume that the problems are all a consequence of a digestive disorder. Fix the gas, and everyone will be happy. So we take our chances and play formula roulette, searching for the holy grail. But we never find it . . . it doesn't exist. Gas in babies is rarely a formula or digestive problem.

The gas that we see in the baby with reflux and in so many babies carrying the label of colic is a secondary complication of reflux itself. More directly, the gas is from air swallowing. As discussed previously, when feeding is disorganized and chaotic and babies repeatedly break the seal around the nipple, they ingest air. The normal smooth, relaxed suck-suck-breathe pattern of feeding is also disrupted, which further contributes to air-swallowing. This air has nowhere to go but down, and that creates a gas-filled belly. This, in turn, leads to pain, irritability, and crying, which only leads to more air-swallowing. And the cycle goes on until the reflux is either treated or resolves.

As gas makes its way through the intestinal tract, bowel movements may seem pressured or difficult. This is caused by the straining to pass not only stool but large pockets of air. Simethicone drops (such as Mylicon), which typically break up tiny air bubbles, do very little to break the huge air bubbles and cycle of pain that all starts with painful feeding.

4. Chronic Irritability

Chronic irritability is a common symptom in the baby with reflux. As acid washes up into the esophagus and throat repeatedly, the lining of the esophagus can become inflamed. This is called *esophagitis*. And with each subsequent reflux event, a baby will experience chest and throat pain. Because babies can't sit up, loosen their ties, and reach for a bottle of Mylanta, their only option is to cry.

As a general rule, the irritability that comes with esophagitis is worse after meals, during regurgitation, and when lying down (especially when babies are on their backs). Characteristic signs of esophagitis include arching, stiffening of the legs, and head turning. When infants with reflux are in the throes of esophagitis pain, parents sometimes hear the sound of refluxed material passing up into the throat. When this is the only symptom of reflux that a baby exhibits, it is often misunderstood as gas or colic.

5. Discomfort When Lying on the Back

One of the symptoms commonly seen in refluxing babies is discomfort when lying on their backs. Like turtles, these babies don't like to be on their backs. Tummy time seems to be better

---

REFLUX REALITY

"If They Like the Sound of the Vacuum Cleaner, It's Colic"

False. This particular affinity was once thought to be the exclusive trademark of colic. Many babies experiencing discomfort, whether from reflux esophagitis or an ear infection, are often soothed by neutralizing background noises. A baby's response to soothing white noise says nothing about *why* a baby may be fussy.

---

tolerated, and vertical time is typically preferred best of all. There's a very good anatomic reason for this. The esophagus connects to the stomach closer to the back than to the front. When a child is on her back, this allows for fluid and stomach contents to flow backward to the most dependent position and collect over the LES. As that LES valve opens, which it frequently does in babies, milk and stomach acid can pass freely into the esophagus, causing discomfort and other symptoms.

6. Sleep Disturbance

"Why won't my baby sleep?" This is one of the most frequently asked questions among young parents. Though there are many reasons why a baby may not sleep the way that we think she should, reflux always has to be considered as a potential contributing factor. The problems with reflux and sleeping are typically a function of gravity. When we sleep we are usually horizontal. And horizontal positioning, whether you're an adult or a baby, can make it easier for gastric contents to slosh where they don't belong. This can create pain, from esophagitis or ir-

---

REFLUX REALITY

"If Babies Scream in the Evening, It's Colic"

False. Like the rule of threes, crying between 5 and 7 PM is another of my favorite cockamamie colic criteria. The fact is that everything for babies is a challenge in the late hours of the day. Their little brains, tired from a full day of busy sensory processing, often decompress—babies just fall apart in the evening. Any type of stress to their system, be it fever, reflux, or old-fashioned fatigue, creates a challenge that's harder to cope with later in the day. They're just like some adults who get cranky and whiny when they haven't had their beauty sleep. And remember, temperament has a lot to do with the way babies handle their stress.

---

ritation of the throat and sinuses, which may make a baby miserable. These symptoms might suggest that your baby is suffering with nocturnal reflux:

- Nasal and throat congestion that seems worse at night
- Cough that seems to occur only at night
- Sudden awaking with painful crying ("pin-in-the-foot irritability")
- Hoarse cry in the morning
- Nocturnal awakening with arching that doesn't immediately go away with your presence

Nocturnal awakening can be an important issue later in the first year because this is when a lot of babies naturally begin to awaken in the middle of the night. Developmentally advanced enough to know that they're in the dark by themselves, they cry out of fear and confusion. In most cases, an environment with fuzzy, recognizable stuffed friends and time alone is often enough for most babies to work this out.

But for the parent and pediatrician alike, discerning normal nocturnal awakening from awakening caused by reflux is a real challenge. The key is in some of the symptoms noted on the previous page, especially the pain and the arching that don't seem to resolve on your arrival. With typical behavioral awakening, the appearance of a friendly face and a warm embrace are enough to make everything better. With reflux esophagitis or throat pain from reflux, the unhappiness experienced by your child isn't quick to go away, and your child will show discomfort perhaps with some other sign of throat irritation, such as congestion or a hoarse cry.

7. Chronic Cough and/or Congestion

One of the most frequently overlooked signs of reflux is congestion. Infants with reflux are often described as "noisy" or "congested." The sinuses seem full, and the throat and chest may have that rattle that we associate with infection. Parents frequently take their baby to a pediatrician with complaints of a cold or allergy. And because reflux symptoms may mimic those of a cold or allergy, they're treated as such. But things just don't seem to get better. In fact, not only do the medicines that are used for colds in babies not work for colds but they also can make matters worse. The syrupy, rich consistency of cold preparations can slow stomach emptying and add to a baby's reflux. Similarly, allergy preparations won't do the trick.

BABY JACKSON: SAYING GOOD-BYE TO MUFFINS

It was a brand-new house and the nursery was so clean that we couldn't figure out what Jackson was reacting to. From early on, he suffered with noisy breathing and what seemed like a stuffy nose. We bought one of those ionizing filters for his room and even sent away Muffins, our cat, thinking that he could be allergic to her. After consulting an allergist, we learned that acid reflux was making Jackson stuffy. While his congestion never completely went away with treatment for his reflux, it was so much better, and his disposition improved.

Like every other symptom of reflux, the congestion experienced by these babies occurs as a consequence of stomach contents bathing the back of the throat. Before refluxed material is spit up and out, it passes around the entrance to the windpipe, where it leads to swelling, irritation, and mucus production. This irritation affects the sound and quality of a baby's breathing and crying. And because a baby's throat is so small, it doesn't take much to affect the way air moves through it.

The sinuses, which drain into the pharynx (the upper part of the throat, where the air and food passageways cross), can also be washed with acidic material. They react to this just as they do to allergies or colds, with thickening mucus production. As sinuses drain into the throat in reaction to their irritation, a baby can experience "sinus drip." Often the symptoms of the reflux congestion complex are worse at nighttime, when lying down makes reflux symptoms worse.

CAN BABIES GET ALLERGIES?

Parents probably overstate the importance of environmental allergies in babies, but babies do have allergies. And telling allergy from a cold or reflux can be tricky. Common environmental allergens include dust mites, animal dander, and mold spores. Look for the following symptoms that can suggest allergy in your baby:

- *Clear nasal drainage:* A runny nose from a cold usually lasts no longer than 7 to 10 days. The congestion experienced by infants with reflux typically doesn't lead to a runny nose.
- *Constant poking at the nose*
- *Itchy, red eyes*
- *Dry cough*
- *Dark circles under the eyes:* These are sometimes referred to as allergic shiners.
- *Sneezing:* Young infants with reflux can sneeze, but when they also have some of the symptoms noted above, allergy must be considered.

WHEN DOES REFLUX START?

Reflux may be present at birth, but its symptoms may not be easily recognizable in full-term babies until they are 3 to 6 weeks old. It takes time for infants to get up to the larger feeding volumes necessary to see significant spitting up and irritability. The irritation that comes from acid regurgitation may take time to develop in some babies. Usually by the time a baby

REFLUX REALITY

"If I Have Reflux During Pregnancy, My Baby Will Be at Higher Risk of Reflux"

False. Reflux during pregnancy is a consequence of the mother's distorted upper intestinal anatomy and is unrelated to any reflux the baby may later experience. Because both pregnancy and infantile reflux are so common, they're often falsely associated.

is 2 to 2½ months old, the parents should know what they're in for in terms of their child's reflux symptoms. By this point most babies plateau—they've developed what they're going to have for reflux symptoms. For most parents, this is reassuring, but for those with markedly irritable babies, the thought of a plateau with no hope of improvement can be difficult to handle.

Be sure to see your doctor if your child develops reflux symptoms after 4 months of age. It is very unusual for reflux to begin at such a late age.

THE BUNDLE OF MISERY AND OTHER PATTERNS OF REFLUX

What's so challenging about reflux in infants is the many ways that it shows itself. One baby may spit up 20 times a day and live life with a smile, while another baby may spit up only on occasion, yet scream and arch with the symptoms of acid irritation in the esophagus. Some feed slowly, while others feed with a vengeance for the comfort that feeding brings. And though some grow out of their reflux early in infancy, others continue on into toddlerhood needing special attention.

PREEMIES ARE NOT JUST SMALL BABIES

When it comes to reflux in infants, not all babies are created equal. Acid reflux in premature babies looks different and can create more problems.

As you've learned by this point, babies get reflux so often because their little intestinal tract doesn't push and squeeze the way that it should. With time, this improves. When babies come into the world 5 weeks early, their intestinal tract is that much more immature and that much less willing to move the way that it should. As a consequence, reflux is more common in premature babies than in full-term babies.

Beyond immature motility, another factor that can contribute to acid reflux in premature infants is the presence of lung disease. Strained breathing can create pressure changes that force stomach contents up where they don't belong. And the presence of acid up in the airway of these little babies often exacerbates lung problems through bronchospasm and sometimes aspiration. The reflux–breathing connection is a common concern in this group of babies.

Reflux in premature babies may look different. The ability to sputter, cough, and clear the airway takes the maturity of a term baby. So until babies are closer to term and stuff comes up into the pharynx, their response may be to simply hold their breath, resulting in apnea and sometimes slowing of their heart rate. As one of the more frightening complications of reflux in infancy, this typically warrants treatment and close cardiopulmonary monitoring.

THINGS THAT MAY MAKE YOUR BABY'S REFLUX WORSE

- *Upper respiratory infections:* Nearly every baby with any degree of spitting up will have worse problems when he has a cold. Nasal congestion leads to mouth-breathing, which in turn causes air-swallowing. The postnasal drip that comes with every cold irritates the stomach and influences how it empties.

- *Intestinal infections:* Intestinal infections, particularly viruses, can affect the way the stomach squeezes and empties. Viruses can lead to spasm and abnormal squeezing patterns in addition to increased acid production in some cases.

- *Excessive use of medications:* If your child has been prescribed other medications, the syrupy concentration of these liquids will serve only to irritate the stomach and intensify reflux symptoms.

- *Formula supplements:* If your physician has prescribed calorie supplements for your baby's formula or has recommended concentration of infant formula, these may affect reflux. Whenever we add supplements to formula, it may increase what doctors refer to as the *osmolarity*. A good way to think of osmolarity is as a measure of richness. The more stuff we add to formula, the richer it becomes, and this can make reflux worse.

Why so many ways for reflux to show itself? All of this is due to the fact that reflux is more than one condition. In fact, it is probably the end result of one or a combination of different problems. As you read earlier, problems with stomach emptying, LES pressure, acid production, and esophageal protection create the "ingredients" for infant reflux. Depending on the involvement of those ingredients, every case will look just a bit different. For example, a baby who produces more acid and doesn't clear it out of the esophagus efficiently will likely suffer serious inflammation and pain. But the baby with a normal acid level and nothing more than frequent relaxations of the LES will most likely just spit up a lot.

Finally, all babies are different. The way one child responds to a painful stimulus may be very different from the way another child does. The temperament and personality of a baby as well as the way the adults around them respond to their discomfort will ultimately affect the way their reflux presents itself. But despite this potential for what would seem to be an endless number of presentations for infant reflux, there are some consistent patterns that recur.

The Bundle of Misery

The term *bundle of misery* was used a few years back in a *Washington Post* article featuring a baby with severe reflux. As the term implies, this is the intractable screamer. We're not talking let's-go-for-a-spin-around-the-block fussiness but rather incessant pull-your-hair-out arching, irritability, and screaming. The bundle of misery suffers with unusually painful esophagitis or irritation of the esophagus from acid exposure. For whatever reason, these poor little souls have a more difficult time with infant reflux than other babies do. Their pain comes from the dull burning that goes with acid irritation in the chest. The symptoms of the bundle of misery can be further broken down:

- *Can't sleep:* The bundle of misery has a difficult time sleeping because this usually involves being horizontal. And horizontal positioning, as you recall, helps acid flow where it doesn't belong. These babies have such a profound degree of irritation that even the slightest suggestion of recumbancy is met with the classic squirming, head turning, and arching as if they want to get away from the burning discomfort.

Babies with esophagitis such as this will often have what I call pin-in-the-foot awakening during their sleep time. Parents often report that their baby will be sleeping soundly and then awaken with a bloodcurdling scream, squirm, and arch. Consoling the baby can be difficult. This sudden awakening is in reaction to the pain experienced by a recumbent baby when reflux irritates the esophagus.

- *Feeds continuously but never eats:* Despite starving, the bundle can't sustain a pattern of sucking and swallowing for more than a few seconds before realizing how much it hurts. Once away from the nipple for a few seconds, she remembers how hungry she is and again tries to feed. This pattern of painful indecision leads a baby to swallow gobs and gobs of air. In fact, the bundle swallows so much air that everyone, including the pediatrician, believes the baby is suffering from some sort of digestive problem. Simethicone drops never work because the vast volume of air swallowed by the baby can't possibly be "absorbed" by any kind of medication. The pain of watching one of these babies feed is surpassed only by the pain that the baby experiences.

- *It's not colic:* If anyone actually believes you when you describe the pain that you and your baby suffer with, perhaps you'll come away with a diagnosis of colic—or, as some baby experts have called it, a five-letter word indicating that your physician has no clue as to what's going on. Colic is not a disease but rather a description. It is more of a concept than a condition. Its symptoms of profound, inconsolable irritability in early infancy associated with excess intestinal gas fit perfectly with typical infant reflux. And as with so many babies with reflux, the more severe symptoms can fade or change as the middle of the first year approaches. What's so difficult about the bundle of misery is that pediatricians and parents often won't recognize the problem as reflux.

The Gray-Zone Baby (or the Not-So-Happy Spitter)

I mentioned at the opening of this chapter that reflux disease in infants occurs on a spectrum ranging from minimal to severe. And both extremes are usually easy to identify. I call the babies who fall somewhere between the happy spitter and the baby sick with reflux *gray-zone babies*. These are the babies who aren't sick enough to lose weight or grab the attention of the pediatrician but are sick enough to make parents lose sleep.

This category represents the majority of babies who I see with reflux. They may not be suffering the most, but they're definitely uncomfortable. They are often a little slow to feed, somewhat fussy, moderately gassy, and always look beautiful in the physician's office. These babies fall between the cracks typically because of a failure of the pediatrician to take a complete history or because of the failure of the parents to make themselves completely heard. Sometimes there is resentment on the part of the parents because they think their baby's problems are being overlooked by the physician. The pediatrician may resent the parents for taking time out of her busy schedule to complain about an "obviously healthy baby."

REFLUX REALITY

"Painful Screaming Is Harmful for Babies"

False. Despite a nearly universal concern among the parents of fussy babies, protracted screaming during infancy is not associated with long-term behavior disturbance or brain damage in children. With regard to parents, the only long-term effect is premature aging.

While many gray-zone babies do just fine in the long run, waiting for reflux to go away can be very trying. And not all gray-zone babies do well in the long run. In some, the symptoms worsen over time. Some develop long-term lung problems; others have issues feeding. The gray-zone babies are the sleepers among those with reflux; though they are often overlooked, their symptoms usually warrant some sort of attention.

Sometimes gray-zone babies are overlooked because their symptoms are attributed to some other problem when in fact the cause is reflux. It is often the absence of spitting up or vomiting that leads pediatricians or parents away from considering reflux as a possible contributor to a baby's problem. Silent reflux is "silent" because babies with it lack some of the common symptoms that make determining a diagnosis straightforward.

The gray-zone baby with silent reflux may have nothing more than one or a combination of the following symptoms:

- Congestion
- Irritability
- Hoarseness
- Unexplained cough

- Feeding problems
- Difficult-to-treat wheezing
- Red throat
- Unexplained nighttime awakening
- Failure to grow properly
- Colicky symptoms

The Happy Spitter

The happy spitter is the baby next door who seems to spit up continuously but is no worse for the wear. Happy spitters don't seem to cry or fuss despite what seems to be an endless flow of acidic material from their mouths. They feed like pro wrestlers and spit up like champs. They do a wonderful job of maintaining their weight by adjusting intake for their volume of spitting. While their splendid temperament may never drive anyone to drink, parents may well be driven to the dry cleaners.

So what is it about happy spitters that keeps them from becoming so miserable with their reflux? More than likely, these babies "strip," or clear, their swallowing tubes of refluxed acid before it has the chance to promote irritation. The gastric juices flowing from the stomachs of these unaffected infants may be less irritating than that of other more irritable infants.

An important lesson that physicians have learned from treating thousands of happy spitters is that the number of times a day a healthy baby spits is typically no indication of a problem. Infants such as these may easily spit up 30 to 40 times in a day without ever missing a beat. Parents consistently equate the high number of regurgitation episodes with a serious underlying problem. Though all babies in this position need a thorough history and physical exam by a competent pe-

diatrician, often all that is needed is education for parents to reassure them that nothing sinister is evolving.

Another common concern shared by the parents of happy
spitters is the amount of time after eating that babies will spit
up. Infants with reflux commonly will continue to regurgitate
3 or more hours after their last feed, or "around the clock," as I
have heard countless times. As you may recall, reflux is what
we refer to as a motility disturbance. Early in life, babies may
not experience the normal waves of squeezing that help the
stomach empty. This delay in stomach emptying frequently
leads to spitting up or vomiting hours after eating. While delayed gastric emptying (or gastroparesis, as physicians call it) is
not considered normal, it is common enough that it shouldn't
be cause for concern.

The Baby Who Is Sick with Reflux

Like the happy spitter, the baby who is sick with reflux is typically easy to pick out. He either doesn't do the things that babies are supposed to do (grow) or does things that they're not
supposed to do (stop breathing). These babies' symptoms may
include

- Significant feeding difficulty with failure to gain weight
- Pneumonia or recurrent problems with wheezing
- Apnea, or episodic arrest of breathing early in infancy
- Possible irritability in addition to the above symptoms

Babies who are this sick with reflux usually come to attention
very quickly and come under the care of a pediatric gastroenterologist. They are often admitted to the hospital for evalua-

TEN LESS-THAN-OBVIOUS SIGNS THAT YOUR "COLICKY" BABY MAY HAVE ACID REFLUX

Sometimes the absence of spitting up can make parents and even pediatricians forget about reflux. Here are some signs that should make you suspicious:

- Arches and pulls off of the nipple
- Feeds voraciously
- Seems hungry but requires more than 20 minutes to complete a 3- to 4-ounce bottle
- Feeds better when half asleep
- More frequently irritable after feeds than at any other time
- Screams when put down for diaper changes
- Awakens from sound sleep with bloodcurdling screams
- You "hear" stomach contents being burped up from the stomach into the throat
- Frequently has coarse, noisy breathing that's worse after sleeping
- Constantly hiccups

tion and initiation of treatment. We'll discuss the baby who is sick with reflux in more detail in Chapter 4, "Recognizing the Sick Baby: When It's More Than Just the Spits."

Reflux Patterns Provide a Frame of Reference When Advocating for Your Baby

Familiarizing yourself with these patterns will give you a basis for knowing what to worry about and what not to worry about: The bottom line is that we don't worry about the happy spitter.

GET HELP AND TAKE A BREAK

Don't live a life of quiet desperation. Besides seeing a physician, you need to ask for help and you need to take a break. If you never share the fact that you're at the breaking point, you're unlikely to get the support that you need to keep you from breaking. You owe it to yourself, and most of all, you owe it to your baby.

Tap into all of your resources: Neighbors, friends from your religious group, in-laws, and others who might not otherwise be involved. You'll get a break, but your friends and loved ones will come to understand what you're going through, which is also important.

Get over the guilt that you may feel leaving your baby with someone else and look at it as something that you need to do. Getting help for yourself is one of the most important elements in treating any baby with reflux.

We worry about the baby who is sick with reflux and a bundle of misery. The gray-zone baby should be watched and potentially given more attention, depending on how she's behaving. Your doctor will probably be most concerned with whether your baby is sick. Getting your gray-zone baby with silent reflux the attention she needs can therefore present a challenge.

4

RECOGNIZING THE SICK BABY

When It's More Than Just the Spits

On October 10, 2005, the *Wall Street Journal*'s Health page ran a story titled "The Hidden Dangers of Heartburn." Predictably, as with most stories dealing with reflux, the article talked only about the dangers of reflux in big people. Up until now, we've perpetuated this urban legend that baby reflux is just a laundry problem. But just as for adults, reflux can present some real hidden dangers for babies and small children.

HOW MUCH SPITTING UP IS TOO MUCH?

Parents often obsess over the frequency of their baby's spitting up. "Continuous spitting," spitting "right up until the next feed," and spitting up more than 40 times per day are all complaints that parents bring to the exam room. And many times they are quite put out with their pediatrician's lack of concern over what appears to be a dramatic problem. So how much spitting up is normal?

To answer this question, you have to keep in mind that re-flux is a normal, physiologic event that occurs in all babies. As we've learned, some babies have reflux without ever spitting up, some spit up a little, and some spit up all day long. The problem is that infant reflux isn't a number problem; there are no black-and-white standards, such as heart rate or body tem-perature, telling us when to be concerned. Fifty urps per day or spit-ups occurring 2 or 3 hours after feeding are not necessarily indicators of anything of concern. They indicate nothing more than a baby with slight immaturity of the upper intestinal tract or perhaps an LES that likes to relax a little more than it should. Both of these problems are fixed with time and patience.

These are babies with simple GER, or those who spit up but don't suffer any consequences. What gets physicians' attention is not the number of urps per day but rather the problems that can develop because of continuous spitting up. Problems with feeding, growth, or breathing as a consequence of reflux help us identify those babies with simple reflux from those with re-flux *disease.* So although all babies have some degree of GER, fewer suffer from GERD. What are the indicators that your baby has something more than a simple case of the spits?

SICK CHILDREN WITH REFLUX—
A BREAKDOWN IN THE DEFENSES

What breaks down in your child to subject her to the ravages of the acid reflux that I've told you "all babies have"? Why does one child get ill and another not? The truth is, physicians don't know all the answers to this common question. It proba-bly comes down to a matter of extremes. We know that reflux is a condition that occurs when the LES doesn't do exactly what it should do, the tummy doesn't squeeze as tightly as it should, the esophagus may not strip acid material efficiently, and the bicarbonate found in the saliva doesn't neutralize as it should. When these events occur to some extreme, babies can become sick. So this pathologic reflux, or reflux disease, occurs when your child's physiologic reflux breaks through his body's defenses and creates a sick baby. How that sickness shows itself will depend on a combination of these broken-down defenses.

BREAKING THROUGH THE DEFENSES—
WHAT DOCTORS WORRY ABOUT

There are three kinds of complications of acid reflux in young children that pediatricians worry about:

- Feeding and growth problems
- Breathing problems
- Irritability problems

These issues are what your pediatrician should be thinking about when you bring your baby with reflux in for a visit. While most babies with real reflux problems have complications from one or two of these categories, some can have them from all three. Let's look at the complications of reflux in a little more detail.

Feeding Problems

We learned in Chapter 3, "Seven Signs of Reflux in Your Baby," that one of the most common symptoms of reflux in babies is difficulty with feeding. The pain that comes with chronic acid exposure in the esophagus and throat can create a disorganized pattern of feeding characterized by short bursts of sucking and swallowing, followed by pain and arching from the nipple. In most cases parents can compensate for their baby's dysfunctional feeding by either feeding the baby for as long as it may take or resting the baby and trying again a half hour or hour later. For those babies who prolong the feeding, the consequence is lots of swallowed air and the gas that goes with it.

For the typical gray-zone baby, parents get through by either keeping at it with 60-minute feeding struggles or letting the baby graze, with nearly continuous exposure to the breast or bottle throughout the day. It's the sheer determination of the parents that keeps the gray-zone baby looking so good and so chubby when he appears in the physician's office. ("This baby's normal. I don't see any problem.") Very often the details of a baby's feeding struggles may not surface during a 5-minute checkup. And the first-time parent may not recognize that an hour is too long to feed a 1-month-old baby.

So how can you tell if your child is having feeding difficulty related to reflux? Look for the following telltale signs:

- Your baby seems hungry, but after taking a few sucks, she pulls away, turns her head, and grimaces.
- Your baby is generally fussy and fidgety while feeding.
- Your baby arches her back and stiffens.
- Your baby's feeding is always prolonged.

There can be a lot of variation, but most babies should be able to finish a bottle within 20 minutes. If it takes more than 25 minutes to complete a feed, you should be talking to your pediatrician. There's more on feeding the baby with reflux in Chapter 6, "The Care and Handling of Your Crying, Spitting, Difficult-to-Soothe Baby."

Failure to Thrive

Some babies, despite their parents' determination, can't keep up with their feeding. So what becomes of them? In most cases, they don't grow very well. In pediatric circles, we call this inability to consistently gain weight at a normal rate *failure to thrive* (FTT).

The definition of FTT has less to do with a child's weight at any one point in time than it does with a child's weight gain over a period of time. For example, a child who grows consistently along the tenth percentile through the first year may be considered smaller than 90% of 1-year-olds, but that shouldn't raise concern that anything's wrong. On the other hand, a child who grows at the seventy-fifth percentile through 6 months of age and then fails to gain any weight during the last 6 months of her first year would be considered to have FTT. Both babies may wind up at the same weight on their first birthday, but the second baby's failure to gain any weight over the final several months represents a problem that needs to be evaluated. So FTT has to do with how much weight is gained *over time* rather than how much a baby weighs at any given point.

So how does a baby get FTT? He doesn't. It isn't a disease or isolated condition. FTT describes a pattern of growth that occurs for three reasons:

- *Poor intake:* If you don't get the groceries, you don't put on the fat. Simple enough.

- *Loss of calories:* Children with intestinal disease often lose calories by failing to absorb and metabolize the energy they take in.
- *Increased expenditure of calories:* Chronic diseases of all sorts have a way of eating up calories. A child with severe burns, for example, or rapid breathing from premature lung disease uses up calories that would normally be used for growth.

How does the baby with reflux fit into this? Unfortunately, very nicely, because they can potentially fall into all three of these FTT categories:

- *Babies with reflux often have poor intake:* This is pretty easy to understand because the baby suffering with inflammation in the swallowing tube has pain when she eats.
- *Babies with reflux lose calories when they spit up:* Fat, protein, and vitamins on the burp cloth don't do your child much good. So even for the child with excellent intake, the loss of calories alone can be enough to create a lousy growth curve.
- *Babies with reflux spend lots of time and energy eating:* Whenever a baby takes longer than 20 to 25 minutes to feed, the amount of energy they burn getting that milk cuts into the energy that they derive for growth. For the baby struggling to achieve a minimum intake of milk, a third to half of their waking hours may be spent working for calories.

How do you know if your child is failing to grow as she should? Unfortunately, you'll have to depend on accurate weighing done consistently on a professional-grade infant scale, with weight then plotted on a growth curve. Once plotted, the pattern, or growth velocity, needs the expert interpretation of a pediatrician. The bottom line here is that the monitoring of growth needs to be left to the professionals. But this may not be such a bad thing because the variations in weight that occur from day to day, compounded by the inaccuracy of a budget scale, can make any sleep-deprived, burp cloth–toting parent crazy. Don't try this at home. Look to your pediatrician for help.

Sensory Aversion

Fighting to feed, or painful feeding, even when successful, can come with a cost. Think of the last time you had a really bad sore throat and had to drink water or juice to stay hydrated. Understanding the importance of drinking, you wince as that juice sits on your tongue. You anticipate the intense pain, perhaps extend your neck, grimace, and choke it down. Over the course of a day or two, this painful experience will give you pause about eating and drinking. Fortunately, your pain is limited to a few days.

Now think of your baby, who, in her short life, has known nothing other than painful, disorganized feeding from chronic throat and esophageal irritation. During the first few months of life, it's this anticipation of pain when she feels the nipple in her mouth that can contribute to fighting the breast or bottle. As solids are introduced, food can create a different painful experience that can worsen over time.

The issue with solid food is of particular concern because of what babies need to learn and do during the latter months of their first year. Between 6 and 12 months of age, babies learn to eat, and that's no small feat. The radical new sensations that come along every few weeks as new foods and more advanced textures are introduced challenge an infant's sensory system. Accepting and processing a spoonful of puréed food takes a great deal of practice. As lumps, bumps, slippery food, and crunchy food are added, there are further challenges. If at any point your baby finds her feeding experience negative, she is at risk of not advancing to the next step. The longer an infant goes along in her first year without advancing her textures beyond stage 1 or 2 foods, the worse her anxiety associated with the new experience of lumps and bumps will get. When babies gag, retch, or spit up repeatedly on seeing or feeling these foods, we refer to it as an *oral aversion*.

Oral aversion can be thought of as an anxiety-based response to a texture or sensation that a child is either unaccustomed to or has previously associated with discomfort. The most common sign is choking or gagging with solid textures, although some children will react to any stimulation, including the use of a spoon or even touching around the mouth. In more extreme cases a baby can even begin to gag upon the sight of a bowl or simply being placed in a high chair.

Oral aversion is fairly common among children with reflux. Even among the gray-zone babies and happy spitters whose symptoms may not seem that bad, this will sometimes rear its ugly head as one of the late and quiet effects of gastroesophageal reflux. What do you do with your baby when you can't get her to move on from stage 1 foods?

- *Be sure that your baby's reflux is being properly managed.* Proper treatment can make aversive behavior improve within a matter of weeks. And when it comes to oral aversion, time is of the essence. See Chapter 10, "Reflux Beyond Infancy: What to Do When the Reflux That's Supposed to Have Gone Away Hasn't," for advice on working with your physician.

- *Expose your baby to textures.* If stage 1 food is accepted, add very small amounts of rice cereal to the food over a matter of days to weeks to add texture. Gradual exposure will extinguish the response, assuming that the pain from reflux is controlled.
- *Encourage playing with food.* Consider adding a small portion of textured food to a bowl while your baby is in the high chair. Let him feel it with his own fingers on his own terms. Feeding is a multisensory experience, and compulsive cleanliness can even contribute to an aversion.
- *Don't push the issue.* Forcing your baby to take a food that makes him anxious is going to create a greater behavioral problem. Play by his rules to some extent. If there is a certain finger food that he will eat by himself from the high chair, let him have it. Any exposure is good exposure.
- *Consider therapy.* An experienced pediatric occupational therapist or speech pathologist can provide therapy and recommend exercises for desensitizing a baby's mouth.

Apnea

One of the most frightening complications of reflux in babies is apnea, or in layperson's terms, breath-holding. But as odd as this may sound, it can be a very natural occurrence in many babies. Under normal circumstances, babies can experience what we call *periodic breathing*, an episode of apnea lasting 5 to 10

SIGNS OF ORAL SENSORY AVERSION

- Refusing to put toys or anything into the mouth
- Gagging with solid food
- Gagging when new, advanced textures are introduced
- Gagging at the sight of feeding utensils or placement in a high chair

---

seconds, then spontaneously begin breathing again normally. It happens because of immaturity of the brain stem, which is the part of the brain responsible for setting the pace for "breathe in, breathe out." Like stomach emptying, occasional blips in breathing regulation are all part of being young and not having everything together yet, so we can expect babies to hold their breath under normal circumstances for several seconds at a time. This phenomenon tends to be limited to the first few weeks of life.

Beyond these normal, brief periods of periodic breathing, however, babies can have apnea for other reasons, such as reflux. When something noxious such as food or postnasal drip appears around the entrance of an adult's airway (or *pharynx*), we typically cough or sputter as a means of keeping it out of our windpipe. This is a protective mechanism in physiologically mature people that keeps our airway free and clear for breathing.

Unfortunately, this ability to generate a rousing bellow of air to blow the pharynx clean doesn't exist in young babies, so when things such as acid reflux appear, a newborn protects herself through shutting down, or holding her breath. While it

TALES FROM THE CRIB

Eleven-Month-Old Who Refuses to Take Food with Lumps and Bumps

Presentation

Sam is an 11-month-old who won't eat. His difficulties began early on with irritability and spitting up that responded to the use of Zantac (ranitidine). His spitting up continued but didn't create too much concern—he was characterized as a happy spitter, and as long as he was healthy, his parents could put up with it.

Solids were started when Sam was about 5 months old. He accepted a variety of stage 1 foods without a problem, but as foods with texture were offered when he was about 7 months old, Sam became more difficult to feed. What started out as simple spitting and refusal of his food evolved to gagging when food touched his tongue. His parents thought that it was a phase and decided to go back to stage 1 foods at 8 months. This seemed to fix the problem, and they waited until Sam was 9 months old to offer stage 2 and 3 foods once again. But this time his gagging seemed to be worse than before. His grandparents were of the opinion that Sam was spoiled and needed to know "who was boss." Believing that this actually was a control issue, his parents took more coercive measures, but there was no improvement.

At age 11 months he was referred to a pediatric speech pathologist for assistance with his feeding. Suspecting reflux disease, the speech pathologist asked for input from a pediatric gastroenterologist. By the time Sam was referred for help, his gagging had evolved to the point where it would begin as soon as he was placed in a high chair or caught the sight of a spoon and bowl.

Through all of this, his spitting continued and his only other symptom of reflux was some occasional fussiness at night. And despite his refusal to take lumpy food, Sam had no problems with Saltines and frequently was seen playing with toys in his mouth.

Analysis

Sam has an oral aversion most likely due to reflux. This is a common problem in babies with reflux and is often considered one of the "sleeper" complications. Remember that an oral aversion can be thought of as an anxiety-based response to a texture or sensation that a child is either unaccustomed to or has previously associated with discomfort. Early on, Sam experienced throat pain from reflux that was probably worse with solid food. As time passed and his first birthday neared, his lack of experience with lumpy, bumpy textures made adapting to them all the more difficult. I emphasize that if babies don't develop the capacity to handle solids by late in the first year, it only becomes worse with time.

It's important to note the response by the parents and grandparents in this case. When things don't go as planned, we often like to think that we can simply make them go the way we like. And when it comes to sensory aversion, this is the worst possible approach for parents to take. Force-feeding or coercive measures will only create stress and pressure for a baby and frustration for you. And this approach will compound the problem. Feeding should never be a battle of wills, especially when a baby has a sore esophagus.

In this case, Sam was seen by a pediatric gastroenterologist. His evaluation included some basic blood work and an upper GI series (series of X-rays of the upper intestinal tract) to rule out anatomic problems. He was given an acid-suppression medication, and his parents were given firm instructions to leave Sam alone while he ate. The speech pathologist provided guidance for reintroducing texture to Sam's diet, and in 8 weeks Sam was beginning to eat foods that he previously had never taken. When he was 19 months old, his acid-suppression medication was stopped and no other problems were ever noted.

This case illustrates one of the reasons that we need to watch babies with reflux despite how good they may look on the outside. Oral aversion to textures is sometimes one of the only signs of ongoing reflux, and if it isn't intercepted, it becomes hard to turn around.

can be pretty darned scary for the adult holding the baby, it's a pretty clever protective mechanism that nature's devised.

Apnea that lasts more than 10 or 20 seconds can result in poor oxygen delivery to the body, with resulting skin color change, loss of healthy muscle tone, and a change in consciousness. This is when physicians worry. Under circumstances like this, simple stimulation and repositioning will often jar a baby back to breathing. In the worst-case scenario, cardiopulmonary resuscitation (CPR) is required. But this is the exceptional case, and for most families, the near-miss experience of apnea has resulted in a hospitalization and proper training in basic newborn resuscitation. Fortunately, the chilling potential for apnea due to reflux is usually limited to the first 6 to 8 weeks of life, after which babies tend to have more efficient ways of dealing with noxious stuff in the pharynx.

ARE BABIES WITH REFLUX AT HIGHER RISK FOR SIDS?

You would think with all the choking and sputtering that babies with reflux do, they would be at higher risk of SIDS. Although the medical literature isn't crystal clear on the matter, it doesn't appear that having reflux puts your baby at any special risk for SIDS. In fact, daytime apnea is much more likely to occur in your baby with reflux than apnea while sleeping. There are some researchers who have even gone so far as to suggest that the stimulation, or arousal, that comes with reflux irritation "protects" from SIDS.

One Parent's "Choking" Is Another Parent's "Sputtering"

I don't believe that there's anything trickier for a pediatrician to evaluate than the baby brought in with a complaint of "choking." Here's why:

- *Choking, gagging, sputtering babies typically are described with vague terminology.* Defining what's happening with the baby with reflux can be very difficult for even the most educated parents. It seems that anytime a baby becomes discombobulated by reflux, it's classified as choking because that's the only term that people can think of to describe the experience. But usually the events that babies experience with reflux are scary but not life threatening, despite their parents' description of "choking" or "losing their breath."

- *There are vague consequences.* Choking can run the gamut from entirely inconsequential to life threatening, so every report involving the safety of an infant's airway must be taken seriously and the situation thoroughly assessed.

· *Choking/gagging is an emotional issue.* Anything that appears to be a life-threatening event to a parent is remarkably stressful. Because of this, parents sometimes embellish or overstate a baby's symptoms to make their case in the most dramatic way possible.

· *The symptoms aren't easily fixed.* When a baby's sputtering is benign, coming up with a quick fix that makes everyone happy is difficult. And when a baby appears to be having some sort of truly life-threatening event, the only option is hospital admission with a lengthy evaluation. Even when physicians admit babies to large, prestigious hospitals and put them through the full-court press, it's still sometimes difficult to establish exactly what's going on.

Worry Less About Definitions

It's important to not get hung up on terminology, but to react to babies instead of to definitions. For example, by definition, choking is an obstruction of the airway, with the inability to move air in or out. Gagging, on the other hand, is the heaving that we do to prevent choking when something is headed somewhere it shouldn't go. But understanding how to discriminate one from the other won't help you when your baby is coughing, gasping, and turning a slight shade of crimson. You can call it what you like so long as you're reacting to what you really need to react to.

The main thing to understand about the baby is that episodic choking, sputtering, and gagging is very common and can happen from time to time as your young baby experiences reflux. Figuring out how to handle an unexpected half ounce of formula in the throat can create a mild crisis when you're only 1 month old. It can be pretty scary, but the baby's reaction is usually limited to a few seconds at most. While it may look dramatic, most babies do a miraculous job of pulling themselves together and curtailing anything catastrophic. Experts in this area of work sometimes call this disorganization; I like to call it sputtering. This is the process of babies getting their act together as they clear the stuff that's in their throat. The more immature the baby, the harder it is to "reorganize" himself when milk finds its way to his pharynx. And as we learned a few pages ago, very immature babies don't even have the ability to choke or cough; they protect themselves by holding their breath.

What to Look for and When to Worry

I can attest to the fact that I have never personally seen or heard of a baby dying of reflux, but I can minimize the seriousness of the sputtering baby only to a point. There are circumstances where a baby does need to be evaluated. Look for the following signs of a problem:

- *Change in color:* Though a deep red flush can happen with anyone who coughs a lot, physicians really worry about cyanosis, or the bluish gray tone that occurs when oxygen isn't delivered to the body. Sometimes we refer to this skin color as "blue-jean blue."
- *Change in muscle tone:* Most babies with sputtering will maintain their normal posture or even tighten up a bit as they get it all together. You should take note if they lose their tone or become, as we like to say in the business, "dishrag limp."

- *Change in consciousness:* Look for any sustained change in your baby's state of alertness. Does she close her eyes and become unresponsive? Does she appear to be staring in a daze, unresponsive to normal things such as the presence of your face? Changes in consciousness like this may indicate poor delivery of oxygen to the brain. Physicians would often expect to see other signs of a problem, but this sort of behavior may be the only sign of seizure activity in a young baby.

The baby who appears blue-jean blue and dishrag limp with altered consciousness during her reflux should be evaluated in an emergency room immediately. In most cases, the evaluation will entail hospital admission.

Sneezin' and Wheezin'—the Reflux–Lung Connection

Despite what pediatricians know now, the association between acid reflux and lung disease is something we've been aware of since only about the 1980s. In fact, the evolution of the reflux–lung association serves as a great example of how advances in diagnostic technology have furthered our ability to recognize and treat the complications of acid reflux in children. Without my going into further historical detail, it's sufficient to say that there's been a lot of effort recently put into studying the connection between reflux and the lungs. But we've learned that proving cause and effect in this relationship is very difficult. The problem is that lung disease itself, as well as its treatment, often *causes* reflux, so knowing which came first can be difficult. It's a chicken-and-egg phenomenon. So,

THE SPUTTERING SPITTER: WHAT YOU SHOULD NOTE FOR THE PHYSICIAN

- Are there changes in color, tone, or state of consciousness?
- Does the sputtering occur with feeds or after feeds?
- Does the baby stop breathing?
- How do you help the baby recover?
- Does the baby experience any unusual movements?

unfortunately, there are more questions than answers, especially when it comes to our younger patients.

So what do we know? Reflux can cause babies to wheeze. The tubules that carry air to the deepest levels of the lungs contain rings of muscle that in some children are more sensitive than others and in turn spasm, or clamp down, making it difficult for air to move in or out. As air moves through these smaller tubules, it creates the characteristic whistling sound known as wheezing. We talked about congestion as a common symptom in Chapter 3, "Seven Signs of Reflux in Your Baby," but wheezing is a deeper, more involved problem. The noisy breathing that you hear can represent wheezing in some cases, but most often it is a result of the throat and sinus irritation that infants with reflux often experience.

It's believed that reflux causes bronchospasm through at least two mechanisms:

- *Direct lung irritation:* Small amounts of refluxed material can make its way into the airway, leading to irritation. This is a lot like the irritation that's seen in the esophagus

"I'M AFRAID MILK IS GOING TO GO INTO HER LUNGS"

A common concern for parents of spitters is the potential for milk or formula to go into a baby's lungs, especially when lying down. This concern has grown recently, given the recommendation by the American Academy of Pediatrics that babies sleep on their backs as a means of preventing SIDS.

The flow of milk or refluxed material into the lungs is called *aspiration*, and the reality is that it's remarkably rare in neurologically normal children—that is, children without disabilities involving the brain or the nerves that wire the throat and airway. Babies have a remarkable ability to protect their lungs from the flow of fluid around their windpipe. And as scary as it may seem, the choking, gagging, sputtering, and disorganization actually showcases a baby's ability to protect himself.

when it's exposed to acid. When the airway is inflamed, it has a greater tendency to spasm, making it difficult for air to move in and out.

- *Spasm of the airways from acid in the throat:* Even without the direct exposure of the airway to refluxed material, a child can wheeze. There is a reflexive spasm that can occur in the lungs when the pharynx is tickled with acid. This explains why children with reflux can wheeze despite perfectly intact anatomy that prevents stuff from going in.

How can you tell if your child is wheezing? The signs of wheezing are best judged with something that most parents don't keep in their nursery: a stethoscope. The detection of wheezing requires listening to the flow of air that occurs deep down in a child's chest. But even without a stethoscope, you may notice some symptoms in your baby that suggest bronchospasm:

- Audible wheezing
- Chronic cough in the absence of a cold
- Difficulty feeding and shortness of breath
- Rapid breathing
- "Sucking in" between the ribs. This is referred to as *retractions* and occurs in babies with significant lung disease.

And though X-rays and lung function studies have a role in diagnosing airway disease in children, the physical examination remains one of the most important parts of a child's assessment. One key factor that makes physicians suspect reflux-induced wheezing is the absence of response to typical treatments. Most allergists and pulmonologists (physicians who specialize in treating lung problems) have a good sense of what constitutes a normal response to treatment. And most of these specialists are fortunately now becoming tuned into the reflux–lung connection and making the appropriate referrals to a pediatric gastroenterologist. But even for pediatric gastroenterologists, diagnosing reflux-induced wheezing can be very challenging. Even among the leading experts, there's disagreement of how this elusive complication should be diagnosed and managed. In Chapter 8, "A Parent's Guide to Tests and Studies," we'll discuss some of the diagnostic tools available to physicians for connecting the dots between the gut and the lungs.

Esophagitis: Knowing Your NERD Baby

Esophagitis is the root of what makes the baby with reflux miserable. While the spitting up may be annoying and the sputtering concerning, it's the esophagitis that makes babies cry. This is the bottom-line result of acid injury.

What's esophagitis? In medical lingo, *-itis* at the end of a word suggests inflammation, so esophagitis describes inflammation, or irritation, of the esophagus. In the child with acid reflux, esophagitis occurs from acid exposure in the absence of the proper acid defenses. Remember that a baby's acid defense consists of proper LES tone, esophageal squeezing, and bicarbonate production in the saliva. Infants are exposed to physiologic reflux on a regular basis, and it's these defenses that keep it from becoming a problem.

A strange thing happens when the esophagus becomes unhappy: It stops squeezing the way that it's supposed to squeeze. Like an arthritic elbow that doesn't bend the way it's supposed to bend, the esophagus stops pushing effectively once it gets irritated. This is important in a couple of respects. First, the esophagus becomes less efficient at conducting food to where it's supposed to go. (Remember, the esophagus isn't a mere laundry chute.) Second, the esophagus becomes less efficient at clearing itself from the normal waves of physiologic reflux that come now and then. So the upshot is that swallowing food can become difficult and painful for the infant with advanced esophagitis. Once esophagitis sets in, the esophagus loses its ability to protect itself from normal acid exposure, an effect that only feeds into the problem and creates a cycle. The fact that esophageal inflammation, as well as these pesky secondary effects, requires a little time to set in may explain why some ba-

bies do so well at first and then their condition seems to deteri-
orate at 1 or 2 months of age, a phenomenon described by
many of my patients' parents.

I've listed esophagitis in this chapter on reflux complications, but it's as much a bothersome symptom as a dreaded
complication. In fact, the screaming that most parents describe
is worse than the damage that most physicians see when we
look inside. In most infants, the breakdown in acid defense that
causes babies' symptoms doesn't create a dangerous situation.
When I put an endoscope into some of the most irritable infants, things often appear on the surface to be just fine. In most
babies the injury that comes with acid reflux is limited to a degree that can be seen only under a microscope. Gastroenterologists refer to this kind of reflux injury as nonerosive reflux
disease, or NERD.

So despite their misery, infants can show classic symptoms
of reflux esophagitis without their esophagus ever showing a
trace of irritation to the naked eye, or naked endoscope. How
can that be? In many cases, the unhappy esophagus hasn't been
unhappy long enough to create the classic findings that we
might find in someone old enough to read this book. If you pay
attention to the Nexium commercials on TV, you might think
you have to beat a hasty path to your pediatrician to save your
child from the ravages of an irrevocably burned esophagus. But
though your baby may scream, arch, and make a scene that suggests permanent damage in evolution, there usually isn't permanent damage.

Despite how reassuring the statistics may be, physicians do
see infants in whom the swallowing tube sustains more injury
than one would expect. After a few months of continuous inflammation, the lining of the esophagus can take on an un-

usual appearance, with thickening, linear streaking, and even ulceration. This is referred to as erosive reflux disease. Advanced esophagitis like this tends not to be a problem until later in the first year, although there are exceptions. The greater concern here is for a child's long-term well-being— early childhood and beyond—because this kind of inflammation can lead to scarring. There's more detail in Chapter 10, "Reflux Beyond Infancy," where we'll talk about the long-term effects of unchecked reflux.

So your baby screams like it's going out of style. How can you tell if he has erosive esophagitis? Unfortunately, this is very difficult to do on the basis of a baby's history alone, although it's safe to assume that babies with this type of reflux are the sickest babies with the most protracted courses of illness. Erosive esophagitis in children is an endoscopic diagnosis and therefore requires a gastroenterologist to put your baby to sleep and look around. As a rule, erosive esophagitis involves all of the typical symptoms of reflux esophagitis in infancy, including

- Difficulty ever advancing to new food textures
- Blood, which can have the appearance of coffee grounds, in the vomit
- Esophagitis symptoms that get worse rather than better with time

Vomiting and Spitting: All That Spits Is Not Reflux

Because I've said here that it's okay for a baby to spit up 30 times per day, it's easy to assume that you should be cavalier about spitting, vomiting, and all those things that babies come

SANDIFER'S SYNDROME:
HOW REFLUX STUMPS PHYSICIANS

If you think you have a hard time trying to figure out when to be concerned, you're not alone. Sandifer's syndrome shows us how even the experts can be fooled. As one of the rare presentations of reflux, Sandifer's syndrome makes babies look for all the world as if they're having a seizure. Their symptoms include arching and stiffening of the back and neck, with turning of the head (often to one side) and sometimes twitching. Babies with this unusual problem are often referred to the pediatric neurologist for evaluation, but their issues really lie in the intestinal tract. It is believed that the symptoms of Sandifer's syndrome arise from the pain of esophagitis and the effort of the child to avoid the pain.

up with. If I've come across that way up until this point, this may be a good time to clear things up. Though spitting up is rarely a concern, vomiting can sometimes indicate a problem. And it's up to you, with the help of your pediatrician, to identify when a trip to the office or emergency room is something to consider. Look for the following signs that your baby has more than a simple case of the spits.

Projectile Vomiting
Projectile vomiting is vomiting that shoots or projects from a baby's mouth. In babies 3 to 8 weeks of age, this is characteristic of a condition referred to as *pyloric stenosis*. In pyloric stenosis, the muscle that serves as the exit valve at the bottom of the

stomach becomes thickened. Milk or formula has a difficult time passing from the stomach and is ultimately shot up through the esophagus. Vomiting in pyloric stenosis has been known to project 5 to 6 feet from the mouth of a newborn baby. On occasion, however, a baby can have a forceful vomit if she gags or chokes at just the right time. If this occurs infrequently, it probably isn't anything to worry about.

Depending on the physician who looks after your baby, pyloric stenosis can be diagnosed with either an abdominal ultrasound or a barium contrast study (see Chapter 8, "A Parent's Guide to Tests and Studies").

In looking for the signs of pyloric stenosis,

- Be aware of the baby who seems to be becoming progressively worse rather than better, especially around 1 month of age.
- Watch for vomiting that shoots forcefully from the mouth nearly immediately after the baby eats.
- Be aware of decreases in urine and stool output, signs that more is going out than coming in.

Early on, pyloric stenosis can look just like reflux, so it's important that you keep your eyes and ears open in order to advocate for your baby.

Bilious Vomiting

Vomit that's yellow or neon green usually contains bile. This is almost always a bad thing in babies. Bile is a fluid that's produced by the liver and released into the intestinal tract just beyond the stomach for the digestion of fats. When it's present in a baby's vomit, it can indicate that intestinal contents are backing up into the stomach. The most common reason for bile to back up into a baby's stomach is bowel obstruction due to a congenital anomaly. On occasion, bilious vomiting occurs with a severe viral infection of the intestine. Any baby with bilious vomiting requires immediate medical attention. Intestinal blockage is diagnosed by either a plain X-ray of the abdomen or a barium contrast study.

Coffee Grounds or Blood

In the majority of cases, blood in a baby's spit-up is nothing to worry about, but you should notify your physician immediately if you see blood in her vomit. When blood undergoes partial digestion in the stomach, it takes on a brown, lumpy, curdled appearance that, in vomit, physicians refer to as "coffee-ground emesis." The most common causes of blood in a baby's regurgitation include slight tearing of the lining of the stomach from vomiting and irritation from a viral infection or excessive acid production. And believe it or not, babies actually get ulcers. Fortunately, they tend to heal very quickly, which is why most of us never know about them. Among babies with severe esophagitis, bleeding from esophageal ulceration can drain into the stomach and create coffee-ground emesis.

Among breastfed babies, blood can sometimes be seen in the vomit when Mom has a cracked nipple. This is most often painfully obvious to the mother, although I have been impressed with how much blood can be suckled from a small crack in the skin. Babies who come up with ingested blood usually look remarkably well, which should allay any suspicion that something bad (for the baby, of course) is evolving.

Vomiting Associated with Fever,
Decreased Feeding, or Change in Alertness

Whenever physicians see the combination of vomiting with poor feeding, fever, or strange behavior, the red flags come out. Vomiting can indicate a variety of sinister problems, including metabolic disease, infection, and central nervous system problems. Although the statistics support viral infection as the most common cause of this type of appearance, you should leave nothing to chance and should notify your pediatrician immediately. Remember that babies have very few ways of communicating their problems to us, and those involve their eating and state of alertness.

Despite this lengthy list of complications and consequences that can arise from GER, it remains a pretty benign problem for most babies. The key is to remain vigilant for symptoms of pathologic reflux and prevent it from progressing. This involves being aware of the complications of your baby's reflux and seeking care from someone comfortable with its assessment and treatment.

These guidelines aren't meant to substitute for a proper medical evaluation but rather to offer suggestions about when to worry and when to sit tight. Though I have made this all sound fairly straightforward, you will need to discuss your baby's particular case with your pediatrician. Every child's reflux history plays into the story a little differently.

Unexplained screaming and colicky behavior may once have been passed off as a speed bump of infancy, but we now know that it may be an indicator of underlying problems. And though most of the time reflux in babies can be managed conservatively, parents and physicians alike need to be aware that reflux can evolve beyond a simple laundry problem.

ANEMIA FROM REFLUX?

While anemia is an uncommon complication of acid reflux in infancy, it can develop because of chronic ulceration and bleeding of the esophagus. Children with chronic blood loss from the esophagus are older and have obvious, long-standing symptoms of reflux esophagitis.

WATCHING OUT FOR NUMBER TWO—BOWEL PROBLEMS AND THE IRRITABLE BABY

The word *colic* is derived from a Greek term meaning "of the colon." Maybe those who associated the term with screaming babies in the earlier years were onto the fact that something could be going on in the intestinal tract. And as it turns out, all that screams isn't necessarily reflux; your baby's misery may in fact have a cause further down in the digestive system. Many babies are unhappy because of what they can't do. So we need to spend a little time looking out for number two. It isn't your job to diagnose your baby's condition, but you need to be aware of what's coming and going with your baby.

Constipation

Defining *constipation* can be a real bear. Constipation so often is a problem defined in the eyes of the beholder. Knowing normal and its variations can be very difficult, even for physicians. I always like to tell parents that it's not *how often* babies do it but how *difficult a time* they have doing it.

Let's first talk about how often your baby should be soiling her diaper. Bowel movement frequency in babies depends on a number of variables, with the type of feeding being one of the most important. Breastfed infants initially have more frequent stools than bottle-fed infants, but by 4 months of age, most babies pass an average of two stools a day irrespective of their source of nutrition.

So if your baby has only one stool a day or a stool every other day, would a physician say that he is constipated? Not necessarily. It's important not to get hung up on frequency. Some healthy babies may produce a stool only every few days, but if this isn't a problem for the baby, it shouldn't be a problem for you. I'm often called on to evaluate healthy breastfed infants whose pediatricians are concerned about stools that come only every 1 to 2 weeks. While infrequent stools like this are uncommon in breastfed infants, if it isn't a problem for the baby, then it typically isn't a problem for me.

Now, the baby who produces a stool once a day or every other day that is hard and rocklike must be evaluated. If you've ever been constipated yourself, it isn't hard to understand how pelletlike stools can make your baby miserable. How hard is too hard? Stools that can be picked up and dropped and then make a noise when they hit the changing table are too hard in my book. Babies who suffer with legitimate constipation such as this need close attention and monitoring before reflux is even addressed. Two problems can definitely coexist, but I advocate treating one problem at a time to establish its role in a baby's irritability.

Hard stools must be recognized as one of the most common causes of rectal bleeding in babies. Much as with an episiotomy during a difficult vaginal delivery, big hard things coming out of small holes don't mix, and cuts and fissures of the anus are often the result of constipation. Recognizing this as a problem is important because, as we'll learn in the next chapter, blood in the diaper can be a sign of another very common cause of screaming in babies.

Grunting Baby Syndrome

So what about the baby who grunts, strains, and turns red, only to produce a soft-serve consistency stool? This is where the definitions get tricky, because most pediatric gastroenterologists would not consider this to be a baby suffering with constipation but rather a baby with one of my favorite diagnoses: *grunting baby syndrome.* Some babies will push and strain to the beat of the band, and this can be very difficult for parents to watch. They feel that they have to intervene and help their baby. These babies' mere appearance would seem to be a cry for help.

But having a bowel movement takes a little bit of coordination. And while most people think of defecation as something as simple and natural as breathing, sometimes babies need a little practice. Eliminating stool from the rectal vault requires the coordination of pelvic floor relaxation and abdominal pressure, something that most of us experienced adults take for granted. But when you think about it, there's a little timing and coordination necessary. Babies need time and practice to get this all together, and sometimes they're pushing in the wrong direction. I always like the example of the first-time mom in labor screaming and raving as she works to deliver, while in the next room the mother who relaxes with deep breaths delivers easily, if not with less stress.

Though the temptation among many parents is to help the

WHY DO BABIES POOP WHEN THEY EAT?

Did you ever notice that when your baby eats, she often fills a diaper? Or perhaps nature calls for you after dinner. This is no coincidence. It's a physiologic quirk called the *gastrocolonic reflex*. When the stomach stretches with food, the colon is stimulated to squeeze. And when the colon squeezes, of course, things tend to move down and out. This reflex is more or less pronounced in different babies, and the response appears to be proportional to the amount of fat in the meal and the number of calories consumed.

grunting baby along with suppositories and rectal stimulation, this is actually the worst thing they can do. Babies with grunting baby syndrome need time and space to work things out . . . quite literally. Only through experience will babies learn how to get relief for themselves. When we stimulate a baby's bottom, her muscles undergo a reflexive relaxation, which will often help her. But this stimulation can be habit forming over time. If babies are left alone to resolve this issue, it tends to work itself out over a matter of weeks.

Anal Stenosis

Sometimes babies grunt for a problematic reason. Some babies are born with anuses that aren't quite big enough to get the job done. Physicians refer to this as *anal stenosis*. When babies are born with near complete blockage or underdevelopment of the anal canal, this is referred to as *anal atresia*. Malformations of the anus can occur to varying degrees, which is why you should

TALES FROM THE CRIB

Six-Week-Old Who Screams, Pushes, and Squeezes but Just Can't Seem to Poop

Presentation

Oscar is a 6-week-old who just can't poop. He is a full-term breast-fed baby with no other medical problems whose issues began at about 3 weeks of life when his parents noticed that he was having a hard time having a bowel movement. Everything was great during the first couple of weeks of life, when he enjoyed what seemed to be a bowel movement with nearly each feed.

After 1 month of age, dirty diapers became few and far between, but not because of any lack of effort on Oscar's part. Every day, Oscar would pull his knees up, grunt, push, and turn a subtle shade of purple trying to get his business done. But when he would finally go, the stools were soft and seedy like those of a normal breastfed baby. What had been a pattern of stooling a few times a day had evolved into dirty diapers only every 4 to 5 days. And when he would finally go, he would fill nearly two diapers. It seemed to Oscar's parents that he was becoming more uncomfortable each day that would pass without a bowel movement.

After the parents called the pediatrician's office, a nurse there recommended using a glycerin suppository to help Oscar along. And sure enough, the stimulation that came with the use of a suppository seemed to do the trick. In no time, Oscar was seeing nearly instant relief when trying to produce a stool. His parents continued to give him a suppository whenever they thought he was having a hard time, which was nearly always. Believing that this wasn't an important issue, his parents never mentioned at the 2-month checkup that Oscar was having bowel movements only with stimulation. At 4 months, his pediatrician was concerned about his dependency on stimulation and after a thorough physical exam referred him to see a pediatric gastroenterologist.

Analysis

There are few things as difficult to watch as babies who can't poop. We can see their effort and even feel their pain, but we just can't do it for them. But actually we can. As we've seen in Oscar's case, we can help them, but this is only a short-term bandage and not a long-term fix. In fact, it can create long-term problems.

So what's important about Oscar's history when it comes to constipation? Well, we learn first that he passed his meconium during the first few hours of life, which is a good thing. While delayed passage of meconium may not necessarily mean anything, in some babies it has been associated with conditions such as cystic fibrosis and Hirschsprung's disease. Hirschsprung's disease is a condition in which the nerves necessary for the appropriate coordination of the pooping muscles never quite develop. Children with Hirschsprung's disease typically are sick and can't produce stool from their earliest days, although exceptions exist. Oscar's early "honeymoon" period of normal defecation during the first couple of weeks of life isn't consistent with Hirschsprung's disease.

Oscar's physical exam by his pediatrician included a rectal exam to ensure that his anatomy was okay. Babies are sometimes born with narrow openings in their bottom that can make something as simple as defecation a real chore. As it turns out, everything was open and normal in this case.

Finally, one of the most important pieces of this history is the fact that Oscar's stools have always been soft. Some babies suffer with painful, hard stools that are truly difficult to pass. These babies need treatment to simply soften the stools. As we learned in Oscar's case, hard, pelletlike stools weren't the reason he had a hard time.

All right, then—we know what Oscar doesn't have. So why is he so miserable? He has grunting baby syndrome. A commonly overlooked problem and just as commonly mismanaged, grunting baby syndrome can create real misery for a baby and his parents. Though we all tend to take pooping for granted as something that everyone's born knowing how to do, some babies get lost somewhere along the way. As primitive as it may seem, defecation requires some coordination of pelvic floor relaxation and pushing with the abdominal muscles. And while most babies don't have a problem with this, some newborns can't seem to get it together.

The simple action of tweaking the bottom with a thermometer or suppository works because it causes the sphincter muscles to open reflexively. And when this happens, a baby can poop easily. The problem with this is, as we have seen in Oscar's case, that once babies realize that there's going to be external stimulation to help them, they make no effort to work it out on their own. Rectal stimulation can become habit forming for babies with grunting baby syndrome.

The solution to the grunting baby is to let them grunt. As hard as it may be to watch, the process of learning bottom relaxation at the same time that belly pressure is applied is a critical life skill for all infants. For those parents who have gotten into the seemingly irreversible habit of bottom tweaking, I will usually initiate a weaning protocol to decrease the baby's dependency on his parents. If a baby is stimulated daily, for example, I will recommend increasing the interval to 2 days in between stimulation for about three cycles and then to 3 days, and so on. During this time, the baby will push, grunt, and turn all kinds of colors, but this is a process that will initiate a skill that will carry the child through a lifetime of healthy defecation.

What about the fact that this little guy was breastfed? Aren't all breastfed babies supposed to be perfect? And who ever heard of a constipated breastfed baby? Breastfed babies aren't immune to grunting baby syndrome, especially when parents start down the precarious path of daily stimulation.

consult your physician when your baby appears to have difficulty passing stool. While some problems can be diagnosed with a medical history alone, a thorough assessment includes a rectal exam to ensure that the anus is patent and of an appropriate size. Babies with anal stenosis are treated with either surgery or special catheters that parents pass daily to stretch the opening.

5

MILK PROTEIN ALLERGY

The Other Colic

Aside from acid reflux disease, the most common cause of misery in infancy is milk protein allergy.

It wasn't all that long ago that I sat as a medical resident and listened to the director of pediatrics at one of Houston's county hospitals state that milk allergy in babies didn't exist. This was an otherwise excellent pediatrician whose training and views dated to a time when the technology wasn't available to determine why babies cried. And until recently, the greatest hope that any pediatrician could offer any parent was the ability to cope and survive. Times have changed and my former teacher has retired, but there are still pediatricians who minimize the importance of milk protein allergy in babies and promote antiquated concepts such as colic. We now know that as many as 5% of all babies have some degree of milk protein allergy, and among screaming babies, this rate may be as high as 60%. We've come a long way in a relatively short time.

BABY JAKE: THE OTHER COLIC

Jake was just fussy all the time. He couldn't get comfortable, he didn't feed well, and he seemed to have a hard time pooping even though his poop was soft and runny. We thought it was colic because we thought that's why babies fussed. But our doctor found microscopic blood in his stool and recommended that we try a hypoallergenic formula. After a week or two, he was much better.

GUT REACTIONS

Milk protein allergy is best described as irritation or inflammation that occurs in a baby's intestinal tract in reaction to protein exposure. Milk (and most foods, for that matter) is made up of three major components: protein, fat, and sugar. It's the protein part of the milk that gives allergic babies a problem. These proteins are made up of large chains of amino acids, the building blocks of protein. I like to use the analogy that proteins are like a string of pearls, and the pearls are the amino acids. The body recognizes and reacts to certain sequences of these amino acids and the result is milk protein allergy. Whether a child reacts to a protein is a function of her immune system. If her immune system perceives the protein as a problem, it will recruit white blood cells to the lining of the intestinal tract. These white blood cells release chemicals, making the GI tract red, swollen, and sometimes ulcerated. For your baby, this means pain.

The proteins most often responsible for reactions in babies are those found in cow's milk: casein and whey. You may say to

yourself, *I don't give my child cow's milk.* But the protein used
in standard infant formulas comes from cow's milk. It isn't intact, or whole protein, but it is cow's milk protein nonetheless.
The manufacturers break these proteins down a little, which
makes them easier to digest, but there remain sequences of
protein that can cause difficulty. And even if you breastfeed
your baby, you're not out of the woods. Breastfed infants can
react to proteins found in your milk.

The reaction that's seen to milk protein in infancy is a different type of allergy than one might see in an older child allergic to peanuts or shellfish. In babies, the most significant
symptoms of milk protein allergy occur right in the lining of
the intestine.

THE SYMPTOMS OF MILK PROTEIN ALLERGY IN BABIES

How do you tell if your screaming baby has milk protein allergy? The first thing to keep in mind is that milk protein allergy should be considered in *any* baby with unexplained
screaming and irritability. This is because while most babies
predictably have obvious signs of allergy, some haven't read the
textbook. These atypical infants can have symptoms that masquerade as other things or they may simply be cranky.

More Typical Symptoms

Between 2 and 8 weeks of age, the typical baby with milk allergy shows some combination of the following:

- *Bleeding, whether you see it or not:* Infants with milk protein allergy often have blood-streaked stools. It typically

isn't a large amount of blood, although I've learned that any amount of blood in a baby's diaper is a lot to a concerned parent. But your not seeing blood doesn't mean it isn't there. Many babies with milk allergy have only microscopic bleeding, which represents irritation that hasn't reached the threshold of gross bleeding. This microscopic blood can be detected only with special cards for identifying blood in stool (guaiac cards). Anemia can occur in the sickest babies who bleed a lot over a period of time, but most babies never suffer enough blood loss to even warrant iron supplementation.

- *Mucus production:* The colon, like the vagina, sinuses, and lungs, is a mucus-producing organ. And as you have probably learned over the years, whenever any of these organs become unhappy, they make mucus. When there's a milk protein allergy, parents often describe thick, stringy mucus that bridges the folds of the diaper and mixes with the blood. Sometimes mucus is present without visible bleeding.

- *Cramping and fussy disposition:* Babies with red, ulcerated intestines tend to be a bit on the crabby side. And if you're told long enough that your baby is absolutely normal, you'll wind up crabby as well. Inflammation in the intestinal tract creates spasm and cramping, which is very uncomfortable. And as with any form of colonic irritation, the process of having a bowel movement can cause pain, which babies will react to by crying and pulling up their knees during bowel movements, despite having soft stools.

- *Diarrhea:* Whenever the bowel is unhappy, it doesn't do what it's supposed to do, and diarrhea is often the result. The diarrhea seen in the allergic baby can come from spasms of the intestinal tract, with rapid squeezing and emptying of its contents or from the release of chemicals from inflammatory cells. Inflammation will often lead to the secretion of fluids from the lining of the intestine. Sometimes parents will describe small squirts, or stains, in the diaper throughout the day.

- *Eczema:* Though eczema is commonly described in infants with milk allergy, this symptom is probably over-rated and occurs in only a minority of cases. Eczema describes a condition characterized by patches of scaly, dry skin seen most often on the extremities. Dry weather and excessive bathing can make matters worse. If your baby's eczema is milk induced, you'll notice a marked improvement within 2 to 4 weeks after changing to a hypoallergenic formula. Infants with eczema due to milk allergy tend to have a more intense case of allergic inflammation.

- *Wheezing and congestion:* Like eczema, wheezing and chronic nasal congestion are often described as symptoms of milk allergy, but in most babies they aren't a problem. For most babies the reaction to milk protein occurs at the lining of the intestinal tract and not in other organs. Wheezing and congestion are also seen with reflux, making differentiation of the cause difficult in some babies.

Secondary Reflux, or Not-So-Classic Allergy

If you spend enough time perusing the medical literature, you may see milk allergy in infants described as "allergic colitis." This may be a dated term because it was once believed that when babies had milk allergy, it was limited to the colon. In years past, one of the easiest parts of the intestinal tract to ac-

OTHER CAUSES OF BLOOD IN THE DIAPER

All that bleeds isn't allergy. Here are some other problems that can cause rectal bleeding in babies:

- *Fissure:* A small, often difficult-to-see cut that occurs at the anus from hard stools. When babies bleed from fissures, parents often describe blood on the outside of the stool only.
- *Infection:* Bacteria can cause diarrhea and bleeding, but these babies usually show symptoms of illness.
- *Blood vessel abnormality:* Anomalies such as the strawberry-like blood vessel abnormalities on the skin can occur in the lining of the intestinal tract, where they're more likely to bleed.
- *Swallowed blood:* Babies can swallow blood during delivery or from a cracked nipple during breastfeeding.

cess in a baby was the colon, and when it's the only place you can get to, it's the only place you'll assume there's trouble.

But with the development and widespread use of infant endoscopy (using cameras to root around the tummy), physicians know that allergic inflammation can occur just about anywhere along the intestinal tract. And when it occurs in the stomach, esophagus, or upper small intestine, the symptoms can mimic those of old-fashioned GER. How's that? If you remember back to Chapter 2, "Reflux 101," reflux is a motility or squeezing problem. And under normal circumstances, the stomach squeezes and empties in a very rhythmic, wavelike fashion. When it becomes unhappy, it doesn't squeeze the way it should, and reflux, vomiting, and pain can be the result.

A study published in the journal *Pediatrics* looked at this potential connection between allergy and reflux. The researchers evaluated a group of infants with proven GERD for milk protein allergy. They found that 42% of the infants in the reflux group also had allergy. Remember that in the general population, only about 5% of infants show symptoms of milk allergy. These findings are remarkable in that they suggest allergy may play a larger role in infant reflux than previously thought.

The difficulty comes in differentiating allergy-associated reflux from regular reflux, especially when there aren't any other signs of allergy. For the average physician or even the specialist like me, it sometimes comes down to first treating reflux and then using a hypoallergenic formula if things don't get any better. Endoscopy, though invasive and usually not necessary, can sort things out pretty quickly (see Chapter 8, "A Parent's Guide to Tests and Studies").

Allergic Esophagitis, the Other Esophagitis

Sometimes physicians see screaming, miserable, arching babies with no vomiting and no other evidence of allergy. And when we look inside these babies, we sometimes find allergic inflammation limited to the esophagus. So these babies have esophagitis by definition, but it's due not to acid exposure but to protein exposure. So they'll behave as if they have raging acid pain but their symptoms won't respond to even generous doses of antacid. This is just a variation on the theme of allergy-induced reflux and requires an experienced eye and an open mind to be diagnosed.

MILK ALLERGY KEEPING YOU UP AT NIGHT?

While irritability during sleep is often associated with GER, allergy can do its part. Research published in the journal *Sleep* found that infants with milk protein allergy have difficulty falling asleep and staying asleep.

THE LACTOSE CONSPIRACY

Frequently when I begin discussing milk protein allergy with a family, I'm met with a reassuring nod and look of understanding. "Uncle Joe has this same problem. He can't take anything with lactose." But Uncle Joe's bloating and excessive flatulence with ice cream has nothing to do with your baby's screaming. This is a common source of confusion among parents, grandparents, and even some pediatricians.

Lactose intolerance is a lifelong condition commonly seen starting in school-age children and young adults. It results from the loss of lactase (the enzyme responsible for digesting milk sugar) in the wall of the intestine. Because lactose can't be digested and absorbed properly in these individuals, it passes all the way into the large intestine, where it is fermented by the bacteria that live there. The symptoms of lactose intolerance are gas, bloating, and diarrhea. And despite a striking similarity to what your baby may be experiencing, the symptoms of gas and diarrhea occur in allergic babies for a different reason. Babies with milk protein allergy tolerate lactose just fine.

All right then, so riddle me this: If lactose isn't a problem for babies, why do we see advertisements in the baby magazines for lactose-free formula? That's a darned good question, although the answer probably lies with the "Uncle Joe" phenomenon. That is, every parent in America thinks that their baby has a lactose problem just like them or someone else they know. And if the baby has a lactose problem, it makes sense to give him a lactose-free formula. The bottom line is that market decisions by formula manufacturers often are driven by parental demand and not necessarily by what is physiologically or scientifically sound. Doctors often fuel this misconception by recommending the formula to the cranky parents of cranky babies.

But before we bash the idea of lactose-free formula completely, there may be a role for this type of formula in babies with gastroenteritis, or infections of the intestinal tract. When a child gets bad viral gastroenteritis, the lining of the intestinal tract can become injured. The lining of the intestine contains little microscopic fingers called villi that contain the enzyme responsible for absorbing lactose. When these fingers are damaged, babies will temporarily lose the ability to absorb the milk sugar, which can compound diarrhea. Though the need for lactose restriction after viral gastroenteritis is controversial, it remains common practice among some pediatricians to recommend a lactose-free formula for a couple of weeks after a stomach bug.

ALLERGY AND THE BREASTFED BABY

The screaming breastfed baby presents a unique challenge. If it's not extended family telling a young mother that she's got bad breast milk, it's Madison Avenue telling her that "comfort proteins" found in their formula will make her baby happy.

And because reflux is so commonly overlooked as a cause of infant irritability, breast milk is often the first thing to go.

One popular misconception is that breastfed babies can't develop milk protein allergy. While it may occur less frequently, babies nonetheless can have symptoms of milk allergy—because portions of proteins that you ingest as a breastfeeding mother are absorbed and expressed in your milk. When I discuss this with young mothers, there's often some guilt that somehow their baby is allergic to them or perhaps they've done something wrong. I always try to make it clear in these situations that the baby isn't allergic to Mom but rather certain proteins from her diet.

The treatment for milk protein allergy in the breastfed baby is dietary restriction of the offending proteins. While some lactation consultants will recommend broad, sweeping restrictions, most babies do just fine with the restriction of the milk proteins casein and whey—in other words, don't drink milk or eat milk products like cheese or yogurt. For sicker babies, this may be broadened to include soy protein and other animal proteins but this typically isn't necessary. But you also need to consider your own health. Excessive diet restriction can be almost as dangerous for you as any type of allergy for your baby. Most mothers I work with are willing to do anything for their baby, but good nutrition for you, the mom, has to be considered part of keeping your baby well.

Remember that it takes a few days to clear your milk once you begin a dietary restriction and a further 2 to 3 weeks for intestinal inflammation to begin to improve. One of the most common mistakes made by moms in this situation is to switch the plan or give up too soon when immediate improvement isn't seen.

Sadly, irritable breastfed babies are often taken off of breast milk without proper implementation of a diet restriction or giving it enough time. Just as sad is the refluxing breastfed infant whose condition is misdiagnosed as an allergy and who is then pulled from the breast. The majority of breastfeeding babies with allergy and reflux can continue to breastfeed with the proper management. If you want to continue breastfeeding and you've been told to stop, you might want to get a second opinion from a pediatric gastroenterologist or a pediatrician well versed in lactation medicine.

TESTING 1, 2, 3 . . .

We're nowhere close to having a simple, noninvasive, reliable test for milk allergy in babies, but not to worry. A good physician with the right approach can help you decide whether this is a real possibility for your child.

Most pediatric gastroenterologists consider milk protein allergy a clinical diagnosis—that is, a diagnosis made on a baby's medical history and appearance (or diaper appearance). Most often, testing is considered information that only confirms a suspicion. So besides having a story that sounds like milk allergy, what's your physician looking for?

- *Occult blood in the stool:* If your baby is having obvious bleeding, there is usually no reason to test the stool for blood. However, your physician may want to do it for the record. Blood can often be mistakenly reported as present by young parents who react with alarm to changes in stool appearance that can occur with the introduction of foods or changes in bowel flora. Occult blood testing is done

SUGGESTED FOOD RESTRICTION FOR MOMS
OF BREAST-FED ALLERGIC BABIES

Milk	Cottage cheese	Margarine
Butter	Custard	Deli meats
Half-and-half	Curd	Chocolate
Sour cream	Ghee (clarified butter)	High-protein flour
Yogurt	Nougat	Nondairy creamer
Ice cream	Brown sugar flavoring	Cheese

with special cards referred to as guaiac cards. Stool is placed on the card and brought back to the physician's office, where a special developer is placed on the card. A chemical reaction occurs when blood is present, and the card turns royal blue. Though you may try to find these cards on the Internet, don't try this at home. The interpretation of Hemoccult test results takes a great deal of experience.

· *Testing the stool for infection:* Most babies with a history of bleeding should have a routine stool culture to rule out the possibility of infection. Infection with common bacteria will typically make a child sick with fever and diarrhea, but it should be excluded as a matter of course.

· *Evidence of inflammation in the blood:* A routine blood count might give some information to support allergy as a possibility. Babies with milk protein allergy of any significance often have elevated blood platelet counts. The number of platelets increases in the body when there is inflammation. Your physician may also find an increase of a particular type of white blood cell referred to as an eosinophil. There are a half dozen or so types of white blood cells that course through our body, and the eosinophil is commonly associated with allergy. Despite the fact that blood testing may offer clues like these, it isn't a required test in the allergic baby. In fact, when my suspicion that there's a milk allergy is high and a baby looks well, it isn't part of my evaluation.

- *Blood testing:* Some physicians recommend blood testing for allergy. This is sometimes referred to as RAST testing, and it looks for specific types of antibodies in the blood to common antigens. Antibodies are the things made by the immune system in response to foreign substances, like proteins. We refer to these foreign substances as antigens. Antibodies are the experience, or memory, of the immune system and allow for a more organized attack or reaction when the antigen is seen again. The problem is that the presence of antibodies in the blood tells us little about whether they'll react to a food. In other words, if you were to test me or you, we might find high levels of antibody to chicken or soy even though we may eat these every day without a problem. This is particularly true in the infant with milk protein allergy, because it's unclear how important antibodies are in triggering bowel inflammation. Skin testing may be more reliable but typically isn't done until children are well into toddlerhood.

- *Sigmoidoscopy:* Perhaps the most direct means of telling if the bowel is unhappy is to look at it directly. Pediatric gastroenterologists do this by passing an endoscope into a baby's bottom to look at the colon and take a tissue sample, or biopsy. On biopsy, we find lots of eosinophils, the white blood cell typically associated with allergic inflammation in the bowel. Most babies who come in with symptoms typical of allergy don't require endoscopy, but it is an important, definitive option for the sick baby when we don't know what's going on.

DIETARY THERAPY FOR THE MILK-ALLERGIC BABY

Sometimes the best way to tell if something is creating a problem is to take it away. And in babies with suspected milk protein allergy, this is exactly what we do. Removing intact cow's milk protein serves the role of making baby feel better, as well as confirming a suspicion. In most cases, this is the least invasive and most efficient way to answer the question.

This sounds great—answer the question and make the baby feel better. So how do we do that? Through the use of a hypoallergenic formula, of course. But this is easier said than done, which you may suspect if you've spent any time in your grocer's formula aisle. There are formulas for every occasion. There are formulas for spitting, another for comfort, one to make your baby smarter, and even one that claims to make colicky babies less colicky. Oh, and there's that formula with hormones that has gotten a lot of press recently. If pooping's the problem, there are formulas with high iron, low iron, and just the right amount of iron. There are formulas for babies and formulas for toddlers (do toddlers take formula?) and formulas for babies in between.

How to separate the hype from the hypoallergenic? There are four basic categories of formula, all with different proteins, the stuff that makes babies wail.

FREQUENTLY ENCOUNTERED BRAND-NAME FORMULAS BY CATEGORY

Standard	Enfamil
	Similac
Soy	Prosobee
	Isomil
Partially Hydrolyzed Formulas	Nestlé Good Start
	Enfamil Gentlease
Hypoallergenic	Nutramigen
	Alimentum
Superhypoallergenic	Neocate
	EleCare

Regular Cow's Milk–Based Formula

Standard infant formula is made using cow's milk protein. This creates some confusion for new parents because they're told over and over to never give cow's milk to a baby before her first birthday. The reason for this is that intact, out-of-the-cow milk protein is very irritating to the young human intestinal tract. The amount of protein is appropriate for baby cows, not baby humans. Cow's milk also contains levels of vitamins and minerals that are inappropriate for a baby's sensitive system.

When our friendly formula companies make formula, they break the casein and whey down a bit and add only the amount that a baby needs. While we refer to this as cow's milk–based formula, it's modified in a way that's safe and nutritionally appropriate.

If proteins are like a string of pearls, then in regular formula the protein looks a lot like a necklace that's been cut in two or three pieces. Not quite something you can put around your neck but definitely recognizable as a string of pearls from a necklace. It's these recognizable sequences of amino acids or pearls that your baby's digestive system can recognize as a problem.

Hypoallergenic Formula—Stinky and Pricey

When it comes to creating formulas for the protein-allergic infant, manufacturers go a step or two further with milk protein. It is heated and treated (or hydrolyzed) to break the protein down into smaller chunks. When proteins are broken down, the body doesn't recognize them. These smaller chunks of protein are added to the formula in an amount that equals what a baby should be getting. It's just that it now isn't recognized as a problem.

If you're like a lot of parents I know, you won't give your baby anything without trying it yourself. But unless you savored the sensation of morning sickness, you might want to pass when it comes to this stuff. These formulas stink. The reason is that when proteins are broken down, the loose ends of the protein sequences create an odor. But despite the fact that the odor may resemble that of last week's hamburger in the back of the refrigerator, the majority of babies don't seem to mind.

The preparation of these specialized formulas involves costs that the manufacturer won't let you forget at the grocery cash register. The cost of the standard hypoallergenic formula runs about $350 a month for a typical 4-month-old baby.

GETTING YOUR BABY TO TAKE HYDROLYZED FORMULA

There are experts who claim that babies can't taste, but the foul taste associated with hydrolyzed formulas can create a real problem for some babies who need them but won't take them. Options for this frustrating scenario include adding a drop of vanilla extract or a half packet of NutraSweet sugar substitute to each 3- to 4-ounce bottle. Table sugar should be avoided because it has the potential to cause diarrhea. You should consult with your pediatrician, however, before adding anything to your baby's formula.

Superhypoallergenic Formula

You may have assumed that the sliced and diced proteins found in hypoallergenic formula would magically transform your miserable, screaming baby into a placid cherub suitable for the cover of *Child* magazine. Not so quick. After all is said and done, some 20% of babies with milk allergy treated with casein hydrolysate formulas need something more, because those smaller sequences of protein can cause a problem for some babies. They don't cause a different problem; these babies just don't get better in the way we would expect. They remain miserable or still bleed or still have whatever other symptoms led us to establish the diagnosis to begin with.

In this situation, we are forced to take a more drastic step and use a formula in which the protein is completely broken down. In this case we're talking loose pearls off the string, with no intact protein to create a problem. Sometimes we refer to this as completely hydrolyzed formula. And like the standard hypoallergenic formula, it contains all the ingredients that a baby needs for growth and development, but without a trace of intact protein for immune reactivity. These specialty formulas stink just as much—if not more than—hypoallergenic formulas. Completely hydrolyzed formulas are as hypoallergenic as it gets when it comes to feeding a baby. And for infants who are truly sick from protein allergy, these formulas will nearly always do the trick to heal the inflammation within.

Soy Formula—Do You Feel Lucky?

One of the first impulses for parents with a screaming baby is to reach for soy formula. It sounds all natural and easy to digest. But the role of soy formula in the milk-allergic baby is very misunderstood.

Soy formulas are manufactured with soy protein instead of the cow's milk proteins, casein and whey. There are other differences, such as the fact that they contain sucrose or glucose polymers as their sugar source instead of lactose. But because you've read the earlier part of this chapter about lactose, you're wise to the fact that milk sugar should have little impact on the well-being of your baby.

The real problem with soy formula comes with the belief that it's a reasonable cure for the allergic baby. But *up to 50% of babies who are allergic to cow's milk will react to soy protein in a similar way*, so if you or your pediatrician chooses to treat your allergic baby with soy formula, you should consider it a gamble. This statistic probably explains why soy milk as a treatment is pushed among mothers' groups and misinformed medical providers. There are enough success stories among babies to keep the myth alive.

But the fact that soy doesn't represent the treatment of

choice for allergy doesn't mean that it isn't good stuff. Soy formula represents a fine nutritional alternative to breast milk and standard formula. It happens to be a great option for mothers who can't breastfeed and would like to withhold animal protein from their baby.

I can't finish any discussion of soy formula without mentioning that soy formula is a bit of an oddball in the world of infant nutrition. That's because it really doesn't have an indication. In other words, there's no instance in which a baby really needs to have it. In fact, if you were to survey a pool of infant nutrition experts about the importance of soy formula, you would probably have a hard time finding a whole lot of cheerleaders. Sure, pediatricians prescribe it sometimes during diarrhea illness, but it's unclear whether it's really necessary. There's a rare condition called galactosemia for which its use is warranted, but there are other options available. So why do formula manufacturers make it? This is another good question that ranks up there with the lactose-free formula mystery. Having observed the patterns of soy formula use since the early 1990s, I believe that the demand for its use is driven by providers and parents who feel that it's somehow necessary or helpful to their babies.

SO WHAT DO YOU DO? TREATING YOUR ALLERGIC BABY

Make a Change; Hurry Up and Wait

Okay, so those are our tools; what do we do with them? When faced with a baby with suspected milk protein allergy, the first step is to remove the offending protein. In most babies, this is done by starting right away with a hypoallergenic formula. You don't need to mix it 50:50 or gradually introduce it. Just get rid

FINDING YOUR WHEY

Nestlé manufactures Good Start, a formula containing only whey protein that is partially hydrolyzed. Whey is one of the major proteins found in cow's milk; casein is the other. While it's been suggested that whey hydrolysates may be easier on the insides and empty better from the stomach, it's unclear how much of a difference this really makes when it comes to settling the irritability of milk protein allergy or reflux. I generally consider whey hydrolysates as being somewhere between standard and hypoallergenic formulas, but closer to standard.

of the old formula and jump right in. Then we hurry up and wait. One of the biggest factors undermining the treatment of the screaming baby is impatience, a mistake made by parents and physicians alike. While it's hard to live with a miserable, screaming little baby, understand that constantly changing the course of action in this case can create more confusion than solutions. Improvement can usually be seen in a matter of days, although infants with allergic inflammation may take up to 3 weeks to show significant improvement. Those inflammatory cells and the chemicals that were released into the lining of the intestine take time to wash away, and it can take even longer for the bowel to heal.

Reassess

It's difficult to know when something that you can't see is better. I have found that parents are the best diagnosticians when it comes to assessing gut inflammation in their baby. There are so many subtle changes in a baby's temperament that can be noted by parents that I could never pick up on even with a dozen clinic visits or even the most invasive diagnostic study. For the baby with ongoing symptoms of allergy (bleeding, diarrhea, skin problems), ongoing misery, and the absence of reflux symptoms, we have to then consider that the baby's condition may not be responding to standard hypoallergenic formula. In such cases, I discuss with the family the possibility of either endoscopy to confirm that allergic inflammation is in fact the problem or blind treatment with superhypoallergenic formula. The advantage to looking at the bowel is that we then can confirm a baby's problem. For some parents, this information is important even though it doesn't change what we'll ultimately do. The disadvantage is that it's invasive. I have found that most parents prefer to avoid endoscopy despite its low risk. I will insist on sigmoidoscopy in the infant who is very sick, whose body is not responding in a way that I would expect, or whenever the diagnosis is in question.

"But Doctor, I Still See Some Bleeding"

Sometimes a baby's condition will remarkably improve but there will still be some residual symptoms. One of the common lingering symptoms of allergy is the occasional streak of blood, reported by families after what appears to be successful treatment with a standard hypoallergenic formula. As I said, some babies will continue to react to the smaller chunks of protein found in hypoallergenic formula. Assuming that your baby is generally happy, gaining weight, and feeding well, the presence of occasional blood from mild reactivity isn't anything to get too excited about. At this point, the only other option to make bleeding completely disappear is to consider the use of a superhypoallergenic formula. And many times the expense of treating the parents' anxiety outweighs the medical necessity of a formula change. In the healthy baby with only episodic streaks of blood, say every several days, I'll recommend not changing from a standard hypoallergenic formula. A super-hypoallergenic formula will cost more without offering a measurable benefit for the healthy, happy baby. You should look to your physician for advice as it pertains to your baby's individual case, however.

Formula Roulette: When Is It Medically Appropriate to Change Formula on Your Own?

Parents often sheepishly admit that they've gone ahead and changed their baby's formula without the blessing of their pediatrician. And why not, with all of the available formulas marketed with suggestions of helping your baby? In fact, some desperate parents change formulas almost as often as they change diapers. In my business, we call this formula roulette. The term *roulette* might suggest serious consequences, but the most frequent result of this practice is frustration. The problem arises because most parents don't have the knowledge or background to understand the differences between the formulas, let alone their indications or what to expect as far as change.

It is entirely reasonable to change formulas within a category, such as going from Enfamil to Similac. Even a change to soy formula is okay, but be sure to keep in mind both the truth and the fiction about soy formula. However, when it comes to hypoallergenic formulas, you should probably seek the input of

SOLID ADVICE FOR THE ALLERGIC BABY

Despite what seems to be universal concern among the parents of allergic infants, introducing solid food between 4 and 6 months of age shouldn't create any problem. Allergic reactions to the typical first foods are uncommon. Remember that there's no race to get your baby onto solid food. You can comfortably wait until age 7 months if you or your pediatrician has concerns.

your physician if your baby is anything more than mildly irritable. Rectal bleeding, diarrhea, or marked irritability necessitates close evaluation and follow-up. Though the Internet has evolved as a remarkable resource for those who want to try to treat these conditions on their own, it has sometimes encouraged parents to act beyond their abilities. It's important to understand the difference between an intelligent dietary change and formula roulette, but of course your physician is ultimately responsible for the decisions regarding evaluation and treatment of your baby.

Stoolgazer's Alert—
What You Might See with Different Formulas

One of my most indelible memories as a pediatric gastroenterologist was of the mother who decided to bring a trash bag full of frozen, soiled diapers to her child's visit. Not a diaper pail or tissue basket–sized bag but a Texas-sized trash bag normally used to line a 55-gallon drum or haul grass clippings. For 2 months, this poor woman had catalogued and saved every

DHA—NOT A PROBLEM WITH REFLUX

If you spend any time in the baby aisle at grocery stores, you'll notice that infant formulas are now available with DHA supplementation. For those of you without a doctoral degree in nutritional biochemistry, DHA is docosahexeanoic acid, a fatty acid that helps form the cell structure of such tissues as the retina and brain. As you may guess, this is pretty important. Although a baby receives a great deal of DHA during the last trimester of pregnancy, it is also available to babies through breast milk.

For the nonbreastfed infant, formulas available in the United States began including DHA in 2001. There is evidence to indicate that babies fed DHA-supplemented formulas at the appropriate levels have improved visual and cognitive function that carries into the toddler years.

But extra fatty acid in the formula . . . doesn't that sound like a setup for reflux? Not to worry. There's no evidence that infants fed with DHA-supplemented formulas have more reflux than those fed nonsupplemented formulas. So if you can't breastfeed, be sure to use a DHA-supplemented formula.

soiled diaper, with date, time, stool consistency, color, odor, and the absence or presence of visible blood noted compulsively on the outside. She taped each diaper shut, then cryogenically preserved it in anticipation of her appointment.

Unlike this parent, you don't need to purchase a second freezer for diaper storage to track changes in your baby's health, but you can expect some changes in stool consistency whenever you change his formula. Different formulas use different carbohydrate and fat sources that promote or suppress different bacterial populations in the colon. The result is a change in diaper appearance. Look for some of the following changes with different formulas:

- Breast milk—seedy, yellow, and mustardlike; nearly odorless
- Standard formula—pasty, semiformed
- Soy formula—potential constipation
- Hypoallergenic formula—looser stools, sometimes described as diarrhea
- Superhypoallergenic formula—forest green stools, sometimes mistaken for black stools

Goat's Milk—Not for Babies but Okay for Kids

If there was ever evidence of the desperation felt by the parents of the irritable baby, it would have to be the fact that they're actually willing to implement medieval solutions such as feeding an infant goat's milk. Immunizations, disposable diapers, baby food from a jar? No way, not for my baby! But stuff straight from a barnyard animal—sign me up.

Used for many years as the cure-all for fussy babies, goat's milk was considered easier to digest. Although it does form a softer curd (the cheesy lumps that occur when protein is exposed to acid) in the stomach, its unusual nutrient balance makes it an inappropriate source of nutrition for babies. More specifically, goat's milk is deficient in vitamins B and C, folate, and iron. It contains levels of potassium, sodium, and protein that are too high for a baby's kidneys. It's true that most babies are able to drink goat's milk without showing immediate problems, but the risk of nutritional deficiencies, excessive protein load on the kidneys, and blood electrolyte imbalances make drinking goat's milk risky, especially should your baby ever become dehydrated.

And while we're talking farm animals, what's good for the goose is good for the gander . . . or cow. Just as we don't recommend goat's milk in infancy, whole cow's milk is equally excluded. Its protein and electrolyte composition is similar to that of goat's milk. Both are fine, however, for children after 1 year of age.

When Will This Go Away?

Cow's milk allergy in infancy isn't forever. Whatever it is about the newborn immune system that makes it react to milk protein sorts itself out late in the first year of life. Most miserable babies with a little bleeding who are treated with a standard hypoallergenic formula can try a regular formula again by 8 to 12 months of age. A small percentage of infants with symptoms of typical milk allergy in infancy will go on to develop more extensive allergic symptoms as toddlers and school-aged children. But for most of these children, ice cream at birthday parties and milk on their cereal will never be a problem.

"COULD I HAVE CAUSED THIS?"

Mothers frequently question whether something they did during pregnancy or early breastfeeding induced their baby's milk allergy. There's no evidence that what you did or did not do when carrying your child had anything to do with his subsequent allergic irritability. There is some evidence, however,

TALES FROM THE CRIB

Eight-Week-Old with Profound Irritability, Vomiting, and Poor Response to Medications

Presentation

Beryl is an 8-week-old bundle of misery whose symptoms of screaming and spitting up began when she was about 3 weeks old. What began early on as an occasional burp evolved to full-blown vomiting with every feed—sometimes up to 2 hours after eating. Like her vomiting, her fussiness increased with time until she was never happy. Her fits of screaming would come and go and were characterized by curling up and arching at different times. The only things that seemed to offer any relief were constant motion while being held and the sound of a hair dryer. Whenever Beryl would scream, her brother would hold his ears and scream at a level and pitch to match his sister. Her fits of screaming were relieved only by the sheer exhaustion that inevitably set in after about 90 minutes.

Breastfeeding was abandoned when Beryl was about 1 month old, when she began latching on poorly. Her mom also felt that Beryl wasn't satisfied with the amount of milk being produced. But even after Mom switched Beryl from breast milk to soy formula, the baby was just as slow and difficult to feed. Feeding was characterized by a fidgety inability to sustain a normal pattern of sucking, swallowing, and breathing. She would frequently pull from the nipple and often took 45 minutes to take 3 to 4 ounces. Her parents reported a daily intake of 16 to 18 ounces despite what seemed to be constant feeding.

Beryl's stools were frequent, sometimes explosive, and very

gassy. The parents never noted blood or mucus. Her belly was frequently bloated.

At 1 month of age Beryl was evaluated by her pediatrician, who found only a sleeping baby with a little eczema. He suggested that the problem was "colic" and tried to reassure her mom and dad that things would improve within 4 to 6 weeks. On the parents' insistence that something else be done, he prescribed Zantac (ranitidine) and Reglan (metoclopramide).

By the follow-up visit to the pediatrician 3 weeks later, there was no improvement. In fact, Beryl's symptoms had intensified. She continued to have marked irritability and vomiting. The pediatrician noted poor weight gain since the last visit and the persistence of a rash. Alimentum, a hypoallergenic formula, was started. At this point no one was sleeping, Mom and Dad were at each other's throats, and they'd come to the realization that Beryl would not be able to begin day care in 2 weeks unless things changed dramatically. Grandma insisted that Beryl had colic and suggested a small amount of brandy on the pacifier. Beryl's aunt worked as a receptionist for a chiropractor who assured her that he could make the baby better in three visits. At that point, brandy and massage for everyone involved was starting to look appealing.

Two weeks later, the parents self-referred to me. During the exam, I noted occult blood in Beryl's stool. There had been no change while Beryl drank Alimentum, and her weight had slipped to below the fifth percentile for her age. An upper endoscopy and sigmoidoscopy were performed 3 days later, and all biopsies showed intense inflammation consistent with allergy.

At my recommendation, the parents switched to giving Beryl

Neocate formula, and within a week Beryl's rash had dissipated and her fits of irritability decreased a great deal.

Analysis

This was a typical case of milk protein allergy masquerading as something else. The pediatrician, thinking that nothing would ever make any difference with this child, chose to drop the C bomb. When I saw Beryl, I initially thought reflux and aerophagia, or possibly a problem with the baby's anatomy, given the extent and persistence of her vomiting. Atypical allergy wasn't the first thing on my mind, although the presence of occult blood in the stool was the clue that perhaps something was awry. Blood can come from other sources, such as a badly inflamed esophagus or anal cut from the doctor's rectal exam.

But if Beryl was allergic to milk, why hadn't her condition improved by the time she met me? She had been treated appropriately with Alimentum, a hypoallergenic formula. This is because Beryl was sicker than the average bear and fit into that 20% or so of milk-allergic babies whose condition doesn't improve with standard hypoallergenic formula. This is the danger of simply "treating and trying" without establishing a diagnosis. While endoscopy has a role in the treatment of only a minority of miserable babies, it allowed a diagnosis and definitive course of treatment in Beryl's case. It's interesting to note that, even after 2 weeks, this baby's condition was only improved, not better. Without a firm diagnosis, it's sometimes hard to have the patience to stay the course.

It's too bad that breastfeeding couldn't be salvaged in this case. Though it might have been possible to "rescue" Beryl early on with a restricted maternal diet, the degree of her symptoms along with her slow growth might have made this one of the rare cases where a superhypoallergenic diet was absolutely needed in place of breast milk. Sometimes in these cases, a mother can continue to restrict her diet, pump her breast milk, and store it for use later in the first year once the child's reactivity has quieted down.

Parents frequently resort to alternative and complementary forms of medicine when it comes to treating their babies. Using brandy is more alternative than I'm ever willing to consider, but recommendations like this were common in the 1950s. I occasionally hear parents admit to doing things like this. Regarding acupuncture, aromatherapy, spinal manipulation, and the long list of other things that people can do to your baby, I don't believe that these have any role in the management of reflux disease or milk allergy.

A picky closing note: The failure to gain weight along with the persistence of vomiting probably should have clued one of the physicians to order an upper GI series. This might have shown a congenital defect in the stomach or duodenum. But as it turns out, Beryl did just fine with hypoallergenic formula, and her vomiting ultimately resolved once her intestinal tract healed.

that for babies of mothers who exclude milk, eggs, peanuts, fish, and beef during pregnancy, there is a reduced severity and incidence of eczema when compared with babies of mothers eating an unrestricted diet. For the average mom, this information probably doesn't mean much. But for those families with lots of eczema, it may warrant discussion with your physician.

6

THE CARE AND HANDLING OF YOUR CRYING, SPITTING, DIFFICULT-TO-SOOTHE BABY

Now is probably as good a time as any to let you know the hard, cold reality of reflux, which is that it's hard to stop it. Our only hope is to make the irritation that it brings more tolerable until such a time that it fixes itself. This leads me to **Reflux rule 1: Reflux never sleeps.** You can thicken the formula, hold 'em up straight 24 hours a day, or play formula roulette, but it will still be there. You may not see it, but if you listen closely, you'll hear it. It's there, waiting patiently in the wings until that moment when you've put on your best black chenille sweater. And if you don't see it, you may recognize it only through your untreated baby's scream. Either way, if you don't believe it now, you'll ultimately come to the realization that reflux never sleeps.

Getting used to this idea isn't always easy. I've found that one of the most helpful mechanisms for coping with the problem is a readjustment of expectations. Everything seems to get better once we understand that

- The issues of reflux in infancy are time-limited.
- The likelihood of serious harm to the baby is small.
- There are treatment options that can often make things more tolerable.

With time, most parents will reset what they expect from their baby and their physicians. When this happens, it allows us to focus our attention on the issues that really matter, such as those of the sick baby.

Now this doesn't mean that there isn't anything you can do on your own to help your baby with reflux; it's just that we have to realize that in most cases we're finding ways to live with it and lessen its effects rather than cure it. In Chapter 7, "Medications for Reflux: To Treat or Not to Treat?" we'll talk about the medicines that will get your baby to feeling better. For now, let's talk about some of the simpler, home-brewed ideas that will help you get by.

WHAT, WHEN, AND HOW TO FEED THE BABY WITH REFLUX

We've already learned that reflux is a motility disorder. It stems, in part, from a baby's inefficiency at moving food out of the stomach. We also know that intestinal motility can be affected by how we eat. Foods high in sugar or fat tend to empty much more slowly from the stomach and even through the remainder of the intestinal tract. But with babies, our options are limited when it comes to dietary alterations, with the exception of breastfeeding, which is the best possible nutrition for babies with reflux.

BABY JAROD: OFF BREAST MILK AND STILL MISERABLE

We went back and forth with the pediatrician trying to figure out what was wrong with Jarod. He was nearly 4 weeks old and still not feeding well at the breast. I was exhausted. We finally decided to stop breastfeeding, thinking I wasn't making enough milk for Jarod. And, honestly, I felt like a bad mother, as if I wasn't able to provide for my baby in some way. After I switched him from breast milk to hypoallergenic formula, he still was miserable to feed and seemed hungry all of the time. Nothing seemed to satisfy or settle him. When he was 10 weeks old, we took Jarod to a pediatric gastro-enterologist, who diagnosed his problem as reflux. His irritability decreased. While I regret stopping breastfeeding, I think I feel worse that he went so long in pain.

Is There a Formula That's Better for My Baby with Reflux?

Despite the best efforts of the nutraceutical industry (the folks who make and design foods and infant formulas with added nutrients), there isn't yet any formula available that convincingly lessens reflux symptoms. Now, you will remember from the last chapter that there is a subset of children with reflux whose symptoms are a direct result of milk protein allergy, so consideration of a hypoallergenic formula has some validity in the baby with refluxlike symptoms who is struggling and not getting healthier with medications. If you didn't read Chapter 5, "Milk Protein Allergy: The Other Colic," I suggest that you stop what you're doing and read it now.

Applying Ketchup Theory to Reflux

One of the oldies but goodies when it comes to recommendations for reflux in infancy is thickening formula: Just add a few rice flakes and everything will be just fine. After all, if thick ketchup is tough to get out of the bottle, thick formula should be hard to get out of the stomach.

The addition of cereal to your baby's formula is certainly worth a try, and it may help matters. I've been underwhelmed with the results that it has brought my patients, but for some, it has worked wonders. The medical literature is also not very encouraging as far as the promise of thickened formula to make refluxing babies better. In one study using nuclear scintigraphy (a tool for measuring reflux that we'll learn about in Chapter 8, "A Parent's Guide to Tests and Studies,"), babies fed with regular formula were compared with those fed thickened formula. The babies who were fed thickened formula had just about as much reflux as the other babies but did vomit less. And as I can attest, there's something to be said for this.

But doping up your baby's formula with rice flakes may not create the state of bliss that you imagine. Here are a few things to think about before adding cereal to your baby's bottle:

- *The most expensive ketchup is always the hardest to get onto your fries.* The first issue is getting thickened formula out of the bottle. You have to be careful not to add too much cereal and make the formula the consistency of soft-serve ice cream. I generally recommend 1 teaspoon cereal per ounce of formula or 1 tablespoon cereal per 2 ounces of formula at the very most. Beyond that, or even sometimes with this amount, your baby may have difficulty extracting milk from the nipple. When this happens, the baby's seal is interrupted with squeaking noises that represent air flowing in around the nipple. And as we already know, air swallowing with gas is an issue in the infant with reflux.

Okay, so we get smart and decide to cut a hole in the nipple. This is fine so long as you can get it just right. Making the hole too big can change the dynamics of a nipple that has been designed for a certain flow rate. This can result in too much milk delivery with each suck and potential choking and sputtering. This can lead to gulping and more air swallowing.

- *Beware the dangerous cereal cycle.* If I've seen it once, I've seen it a thousand times. The parents of a happy spitter come to me looking for help, their baby badly constipated. The reflux is getting worse and the baby can't poop. The parents have been pouring on the rice cereal as a means of getting relief. The stools turn to the consistency of marbles. The baby screams mercilessly for hours on end, trying to pass these lead-consistency turds. The nurse at the pediatrician's office suggests adding 2 teaspoons of dark Karo syrup to the formula to fix the constipation. Sounds harmless, right? But the syrup increases the richness, or osmolarity, of the formula, slowing the tummy emptying even more, and the reflux gets worse. The screaming and straining lead to further air swallowing, and the cough-syrup-consistency formula makes the baby sicker. What a tangled web we weave. Bottom line: Cereal can bind up your baby, and if it does, the benefit that you derive from it probably isn't worth the discomfort that your baby will experience. If the addition of cereal seems to help your baby but constipation is a problem, changing cereals may help. A study published in the journal *Clinical Pediatrics* in 2005 found that the substitution of oatmeal for rice cereal resulted in partial or complete resolution of the constipation seen with thickened formula.

- *Added cereal means added calories.* You may notice that babies who have added-cereal diets tend to be big babies. If you were to add, for example, 1 tablespoon of cereal for every 2 ounces of your baby's formula, you would be adding an extra 7 calories to every ounce. Standard formula contains 20 calories in every ounce, so adding this much cereal increases your baby's caloric intake by a full 35%! For the underweight baby, this isn't such a bad thing, but for many babies it can lead to being overweight.

Added-Rice Formulas

If you're willing to consider adding rice to your baby's formula, you might consider the use of an added-rice formula such as Enfamil AR. While real-world success with this formula has varied, a clinical study reported in 1997 showed a decrease in reflux symptoms in children fed added-rice formula. This formula does not contain the extra calories that come with homemade thickened formula, which may be a disadvantage for the baby with poor weight gain or an advantage for the baby prone to excessive calorie intake. Other advantages include the obvious convenience of not having to add those pesky rice flakes to the bottle, improved flow of formula through the nipple, and possibly less constipation.

> ## "MY DOCTOR RECOMMENDS ADDING CEREAL TO THE FORMULA, BUT AREN'T WE SUPPOSED TO WAIT UNTIL OUR BABY IS FOUR MONTHS OLD?"
>
> When physicians speak about "starting solids," we're referring to what parents give on a spoon as a major part of a baby's meal. It's true that cereal is cereal and what's mixed into the bottle is the same as what we put in a bowl, but the difference is the volume, which is not concerning. There's no evidence that thickening formula in the young infant is associated with the later development of allergies.

Overrated Overfeeding

Parents are often the first to be blamed when their babies have reflux: They spit up so much because they're fed so much. And what you hear, of course, is that if you were a good parent and really cared for your baby, none of this would be going on and you would exist in a blissful state of nirvana where all milk stays where it belongs and babies sleep 12 hours a night. But things aren't that simple when it comes to the infant with reflux.

Overfeeding is, in many cases, an overused excuse for either failing to explain the basics of reflux or failing to offer to treat a baby who may need to be treated. Consider the following points:

- *Babies who spit up lose calories and need to feed more frequently.* At first glance it would appear that the baby is spitting up so much because she's feeding so much. You can get into a chicken-and-egg argument, but the bottom line is that frequent feeding is a consequence of a baby's reflux and not the other way around. And while feeding a little less will result in a little less vomit, the resulting misery of an underfed baby typically isn't worth it.

- *Babies may be soothed by feeding.* Many babies with esophagitis may fight feeding, but some are soothed by the comfort that it brings. In some cases, a baby's natural ability to strip and clear esophageal acid is compromised and only feeding will bring relief. You may notice aggressive feeding in these babies.

- *A baby can't take more than his stomach can hold.* Unless your child has a feeding tube in place, it's nearly impossible to overfeed him. Sure, you can try to overfeed, but it usually won't work. Sometimes new parents misinterpret pain cues from babies with allergic colitis or reflux as hunger cues, but parents can learn pretty quickly which is the case. Babies who are hungry get better in a hurry when fed; those with allergic colitis or reflux may get worse. Just be sure that there isn't another explanation for your baby's complaints besides hunger. The bottom line is that babies with reflux are not normal babies and need to be fed on demand. And that's a perfect lead-in to **Reflux rule 2: Babies will take what food they need when they need it.**

How Your Baby Should Feed:
Knowing Normal from Abnormal

Babies take what food they need. But if we let it go at that, it sounds as though we don't have to pay any attention to what's

going on. This isn't the case. You should have some idea of
whether your baby's pattern of feeding is in the ballpark of
normal. Part of my evaluation of any infant is to get a clear
idea of the baby's feeding pattern. It's one of the key indicators
of wellness in a baby. I'm always amazed at the young parents
I interview who, at first questioning, assure me that their
baby's feeding is going well but then, when I inquire about
specifics, tell me that their baby is taking an hour to consume 3
ounces. (If you think that's normal, you definitely have to keep
reading.) So how much should your baby be taking in, and
when should you be concerned that there's a problem?

The Breastfed Baby

Feeding the refluxing breastfed baby can be challenging because we can't count ounces. We must instead rely on certain
signs that your baby is getting enough:

- Breastfed newborns may take up to 45 minutes between
  feeding and dozing to complete a feed during the first few
  weeks of life. This pokey style can be discriminated from
  the laborious feeding of the bundle of misery by comfort
  level. Babies who are adapting to the breast are typically
  comfortable. Their slow feeding rate is a function of
  breast milk letdown, adjustment to mother, and a propen-
  sity for napping in warm, snuggly places. Babies with reflux esophagitis are slow to feed because they spend as
  much time pulling off the nipple in pain as they do latching on, sucking, and swallowing.
- Breastfeeding infants typically feed 8 to 12 times in a 24-
  hour period and produce six to eight wet diapers per day.
  They may initially produce stool with every feed, though

a breastfed infant should produce at least four stools a day during the first month of life. After 1 or 2 months, stool frequency decreases significantly to one to two stools per day. Growth is the ultimate measure of a baby's intake. Frequent weighing may be necessary for your refluxing baby to ensure that she's getting enough breast milk.

- Between the introduction of solid food and your baby's first birthday, she will gradually take in less breast milk.

The Bottle-Fed Baby

- Bottle-fed newborns should feed about every 2½ to 3 hours, marked from the beginning of one feed to the beginning of the next. During the first several days of life, expect feeding volumes of 1 to 2 ounces per feed and daily volumes of 15 ounces or so. By 1 month of age, most babies will take daily volumes of 18 to 22 ounces per day, which works out to about 2½ to 3 ounces per feed, for eight feeds.

- At 2 months of age, your baby will take six to eight feeds per day of approximately 3 to 4 ounces each, for a daily volume of 20 to 28 ounces.

- By age 3 months, your baby will be taking in 25 to 35 ounces per day. This volume will plateau until solids are introduced at 4 to 6 months of age. You will notice that as your baby gets into the middle of his first year, feeds may become less frequent but a little bigger. You may find that your baby is beginning to sleep through the night after age 3 to 4 months.

- Between the introduction of solids and your baby's first birthday, you'll notice a gradual decrease in formula intake. At 1 year of age, a child has an average milk intake of about 22 ounces per day.

This information should give you a ballpark figure of what your baby should be taking in at the various ages. I emphasize that these figures represent ranges and approximations that can vary according to a baby's particular circumstances.

The Speed of the Feed—
a Frequent Clue to Reflux Esophagitis

As important as—perhaps more important than—what a baby takes in is *how* a baby takes it in. Great—your baby's taking in 23 ounces of milk a day at age 10 weeks and her growth seems to be fine. But you're struggling with her on the breast with every feed or she's fighting with the bottle for a full 1 of every 3 hours. Slow, painful feeding is typical of babies with acid reflux. Their pattern is very often one of frustrated indecision: They want to feed because they're so hungry, but efforts at sucking and swallowing are met with pain that causes them to stiffen and pull back, only to realize once again that they're hungry.

Most newborns should be able to complete their feed in 15 to 20 minutes. If feeding requires more than 25 minutes, you might want to bring up the issue with your pediatrician. Discerning normal from abnormal in these cases lies in the details of what your baby is doing. On the breast, for example, cozy surroundings will cause some babies to fall asleep very quickly and require regular stimulation to get them to stick with it and get the job done. When babies are learning to breastfeed during the first couple of weeks, it isn't uncommon for them to take up to 45 minutes to complete feeding from both breasts. This is quite different from the alert, hungry baby desperate to feed but unable to because of discomfort.

**POOR FEEDING: OTHER THINGS TO THINK OF
BESIDES REFLUX**

- Anatomic problems in the mouth and throat
- Thrush (a fungal disease)
- Ear or throat infection
- Teething
- Constipation
- Foreign object in the esophagus

No Baby Should Be Forced to Live by the Clock

We can see that even among healthy babies, there's a range of normal patterns of intake. And when we factor in esophagitis, the pattern can become more difficult to discern. As we've learned, infants suffering with reflux can have marginal intake and, in turn, can require frequent feeding to maintain hydration and growth. All of this means that schedules are difficult under normal circumstances and can be downright dangerous for babies with reflux.

But if you read plenty of parenting books, you'll get the impression that everything will be rosy if you just stick to a schedule. The book *Babywise*, for example, advocates what it refers to as parent directed feeding. The basis of this philosophy is that babies are incapable of regulating their intake and that it must be you, the parent, who establishes "hunger patterns." In other words, you should determine what works best for you so as not to cut into your 9 A.M. spinning class. And the authors warn ominously that a failure to control children when they're young will result in further difficulties when they're preteens and teenagers. The authors even suggest that a baby shouldn't be allowed to hold a bottle because that would mean that you have relinquished control that you alone should maintain.

I've found that the strict regimentation suggested in books such as *Babywise* appeals to those parents who strive for complete control—and often these are the parents who feel most out of control. But strict scheduling should be avoided, especially in babies whose underlying medical conditions prevent them from doing exactly what's convenient for their parents. In fact, this pattern of feeding, beyond prolonging your baby's suffering, may be dangerous. Infants with reflux, for example, will lose calories when they spit up or may not take adequate calories at any given feed. They will in turn need to feed sooner to make up for what they didn't get earlier. If they are denied this, they're at risk for poor growth and dehydration.

Breastfeeding the Infant with Reflux

If there ever were a time when schedules were contraindicated for a child's health and well-being, it would have to be during the early weeks of breastfeeding. One of the most important factors contributing to the successful development of a healthy milk supply is frequent breast stimulation by feeding and bonding early in a baby's life. During the first few weeks of life, breastfeeding may be marked by frequent, protracted feeds that mix at times with napping. Ultimately, your production of milk will begin to meet your baby's needs. And just when you think you have it down, your baby may experience a growth spurt and demand feeding more frequently than every 3 to 4 hours. Schedules and breastfeeding just don't mix. When you

REFLUX REALITY

"Babies Scream Because Their Parents Spoil Them and Don't Set Limits and Schedules"

False. Like feeding schedules, rigid policies should be avoided that dictate that a baby scream as a means of learning to quiet herself. Failing to pay attention to the baby who screams as a means of expressing her pain is irresponsible. Newborns cannot be spoiled and need nurturing to feel secure.

observe mothers who breastfeed successfully, they establish a natural give-and-take pattern that's flexible enough to work for them and their babies.

The issues facing the breastfeeding infant with reflux are really no different from those of the baby who feeds from a bottle, although I should say that there's a lot more at stake. When you talk to lactation consultants or physicians who study the patterns of breastfeeding, they will sometimes refer to what are called breastfeeding roadblocks, or pitfalls, that cause mothers to never begin breastfeeding or stop breastfeeding when things aren't going as well as planned. Common roadblocks include false preconceived notions about breastfeeding, cracked nipples, and the belief that you're not producing enough milk.

There's more at stake for the breastfeeding baby because once you stop breastfeeding, it's difficult to restart without a lot of hard work. And when a baby has difficulty feeding from acid reflux, the first impulse of mothers can be to ditch the breast and go to bottle-feeding—and even some physicians advise this. Many times it isn't clear why a baby is arching and pulling away from the nipple or screaming after feeds. With the frequent feeding often required by the baby with reflux, the perception may be that the baby isn't getting what she needs. But as we've learned, this is typical behavior of the infant with reflux. Also, making the change to bottle-feeding is often the worst thing that a desperate mother can do, because breast milk is absolutely the best nutritional substrate for the infant with reflux. Despite the fact that the formula manufacturers have sought reflux solutions, nothing they produce matches the qualities of breast milk as far as helping your baby with reflux: Breast milk empties very efficiently from the stomach, compared with formula, and impaired stomach emptying is one of the major factors contributing to reflux in infancy. A study reported in 1992 in the *Journal of Pediatric Gastroenterology and Nutrition* compared full-term babies fed formula with those fed breast milk to evaluate reflux during sleep during the first week of life. The researchers found that the formula-fed babies had more reflux than their breastfed counterparts. Factor in that breast milk doesn't stain, that it has a faintly pleasant odor that's barely detectable compared with that of most formulas, that the poops of newborns who receive only breast milk don't stink the way formula-fed babies' poops do, and that breast milk costs nothing and requires no mixing and heating, and it's a no-brainer.

Weaned Babies Reflux More

If you don't believe that breast milk has a significant impact on naturally controlling baby's reflux, you can prove it by talking to some of your working-mother friends. Find one who has a baby with reflux who weaned from the breast so that the mother could return to work. I can predict with some certainty that she will have noticed some increase in her baby's reflux symptoms with the change to formula. I've seen this in my practice on countless occasions and I regularly warn soon-to-be working mothers of my **Reflux rule 3: Weaned babies reflux more than breastfeeding babies.** The increase in reflux that you notice shouldn't be enough to alter your life plans significantly. But if your baby is a gray-zone baby or has significant disease, it could have an impact on her health. For happy spitters and the gray-zone baby with fewer problems, weaning from the breast shouldn't result in anything more than an increase in wet burps.

Should Breastfeeding Mothers Eat Differently When Their Child Has Gastroesophageal Reflux Disease?

Breastfeeding mothers almost universally alter their diet whenever their baby's health is anything other than perfect. It's a built-in cultural understanding that if your baby is irritable, it must be something you're doing or not doing that's to blame.

In the previous chapter we saw that about 5% of all babies have some degree of milk protein hypersensitivity. Such proteins find their way into your breast milk and can wreak havoc just like the proteins found in bottled formula. And while many babies with allergy will show some evidence of intestinal irritation with bleeding or eczema, or even refluxlike symptoms when the allergic inflammation hits the upper intestinal tract, some will show nothing more than otherwise unexplainable fussy behavior.

So it is entirely reasonable to withhold foods containing casein and whey if your baby has experienced unusual, unexplainable fussiness. In the previous chapter, I offered some guidelines for protein restriction in the breastfeeding mother. Remember that it will take a couple of days to clear your breast milk of offending proteins and up to 3 weeks for your baby's intestinal tract to heal, so be patient and don't expect overnight changes.

Beyond proteins that can create irritability in your baby, there are the foods that the playgroup crowd warns against. Foods that give some of us adults gas, such as broccoli and cauliflower, are touted as gas forming for babies, although I'm unaware of any controlled clinical studies showing their influence on how often babies break wind. I have, however, had numerous intelligent, observant mothers report to me that spicy items such as marinara sauce and curry have clear effects on the esophagitis symptoms their refluxing baby experienced. And there may be something to this, because we know that the flavors experienced by breastfeeding babies vary widely because of the various foods that their mothers eat. Proven guidelines in this very gray area of lactation medicine are hard to come by, so my advice is for you to experiment on your own and avoid spicy, highly seasoned foods.

A Word About Bottles, Nipples, and Other Feeding Paraphernalia

Next to formulas, one of the pillars of the cottage industry spawned by the irritable baby is feeding paraphernalia. And it seems there are as many bottle systems as there are formulas. Most employ some cockamamie double-talk for minimizing gas and maximizing happiness. Having treated thousands of babies labeled with the C word, I have found that most have run the gamut of the popular bottle systems and failed to find significant relief. There's a very good reason for this: Bottles don't fix reflux. The bottle is nothing more than a reservoir for holding milk until such a time that it can flow into the nipple for expression and swallowing. Assuming that you don't shake your baby's bottle as if you're mixing a martini, there's little that this reservoir can do to minimize gas. Bubbles in your baby's bottle should rise to the back of the bottle and never see the digestive tract if the bottle is held properly.

But nipples do make a difference, and this is what you should be paying attention to. Every baby has slightly different anatomy, so feeding efficiency can be influenced by the shape and compressibility of a nipple. A nipple that's too hard will be difficult to pull milk from. A nipple that's too soft will collapse when a baby begins to suck. In both cases, you will notice lots of squeaking and squawking noises as air escapes in around the nipple—and gets swallowed. The right fit will result in a relaxed suck-suck-swallow-breathe pattern that's rhythmic and relatively quiet. When you listen to your baby feed, you should hear only swallowing and breathing. While you may need to shop around to find what works best for your baby, the Avent bottle system is one of my favorites. Their products emphasize the nipple as one of the most important variables in a bottle system.

But despite your best intentions for finding that perfect nipple, the baby with acid reflux may struggle no matter how many you try. In this instance, the baby's symptoms of esophagitis must be treated to establish some order in her feedings.

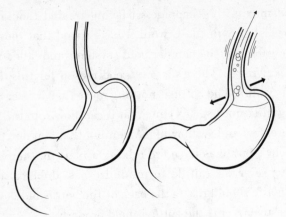

THE ANATOMY OF A BURP

A successful burp requires that stomach air be positioned near the lower esophageal sphincter at the time it relaxes. This requires patience, positioning, and a little bit of luck.

Taking a Position on Burping

Parents are quick to blame gas on a baby's formula, but the reality is that most cases of painful gas are caused by swallowed air. And the first and best means of avoiding gas in a baby is to prevent it. The second best means of avoiding painful gas is to get rid of it once it gets to the stomach. This is probably as good a time as any to discuss a little bit about the basics of burping. Knowing the how and why of burping in a baby helps us understand the baby who's hard to burp and the relationship between burping and reflux.

As we already know, babies have a habit of swallowing air when they feed. Under normal circumstances in a baby who is held upright, air will accumulate in the fundus, or dome of the stomach. To help a baby do what she can't do herself, we en-

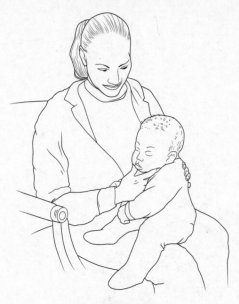

THE PALM BURP

gage in a ritual that facilitates the freeing of that air so that it doesn't cause pain and problems later on—burping the baby. Burping occurs when that bubble of air in the fundus moves near the LES at around the time that the LES undergoes one of its *transient relaxations*. In other words, it opens up quite frequently as one of the physiologic quirks that leads babies to have as much reflux as they do. With all of our tricks to get a baby to burp, we are doing nothing more than helping that air position itself in just the right place and patiently waiting for nature to offer up an LES relaxation. The ability to burp is mostly a function of a baby's anatomy but often is a function of the experience and skill of the burper. Some of the most difficult-to-burp babies (even in the hands of an experienced

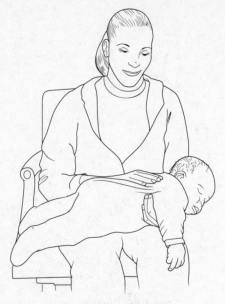

THE LAP BURP

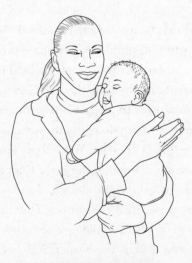

THE SHOULDER BURP

STIRRED, NOT SHAKEN

Agent 007 preferred his drinks "shaken, not stirred," but you should never shake powdered formula to mix it up. This puts air bubbles into the formula that will ultimately wreak havoc in your baby's intestinal tract. But if you *must* shake, allow the bottle to sit for at least 15 to 20 minutes to allow bubbles to rise and pop. If time is of the essence, stir gently until the formula is well mixed.

burper) are that way because of the shape of their stomachs and the pattern of their LES relaxation.

Popular wisdom dictates that the baby with reflux should be burped frequently. This is probably because we know that air swallowing is a common issue in this group of babies. But keep in mind that burping a baby probably does more to prevent gas than it does to change the course of an infant's reflux. Interrupting feeds to burp can be hard, especially when a baby doesn't want to be interrupted. For some babies with reflux, burping can be painful because some acid comes up with the burp. But despite its potential shortcomings, burping every ounce and a half is probably a good preventive measure against swallowed air.

The Empty Promise of Solid Food: Dirty Harry and the Rule of Thirds

One of the current myths about babies and reflux is that the introduction of solid foods leads to improvement. I wish that there were a magic process of starting solids for the baby with

PACIFIERS AND THE BABY WITH REFLUX

A pacifier may soothe your fussy baby, but probably not because it helps her reflux. Studies looking at this issue have failed to show any convincing evidence that pacifiers reduce acid reflux symptoms in babies.

reflux—it would not only help babies but also empower parents and give magazine editors fodder for articles on how simple it is for busy working mothers to make their spitter better with "three easy steps." But, unfortunately, I'm stuck bearing the bad news that solid food is probably overrated when it comes to reversing the reflux curse.

If we once again apply the ketchup theory to reflux, we would assume that thickening what we send to our babies' stomachs can only help matters. (Remember, expensive ketchup is harder to get out of the bottle than cheap ketchup.) For some babies, this is the case, but for others, it makes no difference. Reports of studies looking at the impact of different kinds of food on different kinds of babies are hard to come by, so I'm forced to rely on my personal experience. And my experience has been that about a third of babies with reflux show no change after the start of solids, a third get better, and a third get worse. I use this *rule of thirds* illustration with families as a gentle means of letting them know that solids are a bit of a crap shoot when it comes to acid reflux. Or in the words of Clint Eastwood as Dirty Harry, "Do you feel lucky?"

Irrespective of what you see or hear as far as success stories, keep in mind that solid foods are often started during a period

HOW TO HANDLE THE BABY WHO WON'T BURP

Can't get your baby to burp? Here are a couple of things to keep in mind:

- *Maybe he doesn't need to.* Some babies don't take in much air or burp quietly. While most babies need to be burped, he may not be like the baby next door.
- *Change positions.* Remember that burping is a function of anatomy. Change positions to find what works for your baby.
- *Be persistent.* It may take 2 to 3 minutes to elicit a burp. Don't give up too soon.
- *Don't be rigid.* Depending on the temperament of your baby, time away from the nipple may create a crisis that gets him more worked up than relieved. If you've tried three positions and given it 3 minutes, consider moving on.

of peak natural improvement in reflux symptoms. My recommendation would be not to let it become a preoccupation and feed your baby as you normally would. Here are a few things to keep in mind:

- *The type of food doesn't matter.* There's a whole lot of advice about foods to avoid in babies with reflux, but it's nothing more than folklore. There's the urban legend that dictates that vegetables should be started before fruits to avoid the dreaded sweet tooth, and then there's the one that says that fruits may not be as well tolerated by the baby with reflux. But the concentration, or osmolarity, of a food or formula—which is what truly affects stomach emptying—varies very little among the first foods given to babies. I'm not aware of any stage 1 foods that should be avoided in the refluxing baby.

So what about the introduction of more advanced foods or the early introduction of table food? The advice really isn't any different. The foods that are generally sold as stage 2 or 3 baby foods don't represent nutritional extremes that are likely to cause a problem. When it comes to table food, rich, heavily seasoned food should be avoided. That includes foods with cream sauces or cheese. Simple foods such as plain, overcooked pasta and soft-cooked vegetables make great choices. And if all goes well, by late in the first year, reflux should evolve to become less of an issue rather than one that warrants a special diet.

- *You can start giving solids at the normal time.* Solid food in the baby with reflux can be started at 4 to 6 months of age, just as with any other baby. But keep in mind that this isn't a race, and as I hope I've made clear, there's no evidence that this is going to make your baby's reflux miraculously disappear.

- *More spitting doesn't mean put the spoon away.* Be prepared for the likelihood that your baby's reflux will pick up a bit after the introduction of solids, but this isn't an indication that solids need to be stopped. In fact, the oral stimulation that babies receive from their solid food is an important part of their learning to swallow foods. Solids have the potential to create more of a mess, but their impact on your baby's intestinal health probably doesn't amount to much.

- *Be prepared for solids to be gagged on, refused, or pushed away.* For those of you who have had the experience of starting a baby on solid food, you may have found that things don't always turn out like the baby food advertisement where the giggling cherub willfully accepts whatever Mom or Dad delivers. Handling solid food is one of many experiences babies are slow to pick up on. In fact, before age 4 months or so, babies have a built-in mechanism that protects them from trying to take in things that their anatomy isn't yet prepared for—the *extrusor reflex*. This is the mostly annoying but sometimes cute response of babies during those early days of feeding: The mouth opens a bit and food easily goes in, and just as you've started the video recorder, out comes the food, with the tongue not far behind. This is acceptable behavior for early feeding and doesn't suggest that anything's awry. You'll find that after a week or two of such experiences your baby will, by chance, discover the pleasure of having a little food leak to the back of the tongue. Lo and behold, she's forming a little bolus, swallowing, and looking for more.

For most babies with reflux, this will be the case. Be aware, however, that just as there are babies who winced and pulled away from the bottle early on, there will be babies who will wince and gag at the sensation of solid food in the throat. An occasional cough and sputter is acceptable, but the baby who consistently gags when solids are introduced requires special care. This is something that should be closely monitored by your pediatrician, but many times consultation with a pediatric gastroenterologist is necessary.

This is what a physician will do for the baby with reflux who gags or consistently refuses food:

THE EXTRUSOR REFLEX

The ability for a baby to handle food is acquired after approximately 4 months of age. Before that time the muscles and nerves required to organize food into a bolus aren't coordinated enough to allow for safe, efficient eating, so as a means of preventing choking or gagging, babies have what is referred to as an extrusor reflex. This is the tongue thrust that parents witness when first giving solids to their baby. When the baby detects solid food on his tongue, he pushes it out onto a bib instead of pushing it to the back of his mouth.

- *The first order of business is to establish that there's nothing mechanical that could be interfering with the passage of solid food from the tongue to the stomach.* This is often done with an upper GI series, which you will read about in Chapter 8, "A Parent's Guide to Tests and Studies." Depending on the details of what a baby is or isn't doing with her food, a swallow study with a pediatric speech pathologist may be indicated to rule out the possibility that food is sneaking into the lungs.

- *We next want to make sure that her reflux is under adequate control.* One of the early signs of evolving esophagitis is refusal to take solid food. Painful swallowing, when repeated, will create an experience that a baby will begin to associate with the sensation of food on the tongue. Once this behavior is learned, it is an *oral aversion.* Oral aversion due to reflux in infancy typically improves with therapy by an experienced feeding therapist.

• *Once reflux is treated, we want to be very careful with how we feed.* Continued exposure to food in the baby who has learned that swallowing will be painful could potentially make matters worse, so be sure to get expert advice from a gastroenterologist or other feeding specialist. When a baby is on her way to recovery from reflux, very runny food or cereal is used to get her comfortable with texture. And as time goes on, lumps and bumps are added as the baby can tolerate them. I often recommend simple protocols like this in mild cases. In more serious cases of aversion, especially in babies late in the first year, I'll provide a referral to a pediatric occupational therapist or speech pathologist.

Good Table Foods for Your Refluxing Baby

Be prepared: Your baby's refusal to eat his puréed "ham and liver dinner" may represent his dawning realization of what he's actually eating. And often, by 8 to 9 months of age, your baby will begin eyeing the colors and shapes on your own plate. When he begins to realize that there are options, don't be surprised to see the characteristic head turn and arch indicating that he knows what's in that jar. At that point, it's entirely reasonable to begin to let him sample what you've got or even include him in the meal. Stick to soft, easy-to-gum foods. Remember that babies don't necessarily need teeth to begin eating table food. During the second half of your baby's first year, he should develop the ability to pick something off the high chair tray with a scissor or pincer grasp.

As far as his reflux is concerned, be aware that textures could be an issue, but that should not stop you from trying. If you notice that advanced-texture foods are gagged, don't push them. You might downshift to the baby food he tolerates and try again in 2 weeks. Otherwise, as mentioned earlier, stay away from rich, heavy foods or those that are seasoned or spiced. Here are some good options for finger foods for the refluxing baby, or any baby, late in infancy:

- Cooked fusilli without sauce
- Small pancakes
- Diced canned peaches
- Cheerios
- Elbow macaroni
- Cooked carrots, sliced and quartered
- Banana slices
- Cooked green beans

TAKING A POSITION ON REFLUX—PUTTING GRAVITY ON YOUR SIDE

Remember that no matter what we talk about in this book as far as diet, medicines, or surgery, treating reflux comes down to keeping inside the baby what goes into the baby. And when it comes to achieving this goal, gravity must be considered. But positioning, like feeding, may be overrated in reversing the reflux curse. In fact, keeping a baby in a position that prevents reflux to any significant degree may be close to impossible. And here's why:

- *Babies move.* For the few weeks that a baby's mobility is limited, keeping her where you want her is easy. But once she gets to rolling and crawling, it's hard to keep a healthy baby down . . . or up, in this case.

- *Babies ultimately are horizontal creatures.* You can hold them and you can prop them, but no matter how hard we work at it, they ultimately wind up in a position most conducive to reflux: horizontal.
- *Babies reflux all the time.* Remember that all babies have reflux and babies are always refluxing, whether we see it or not. Maintaining vertical posture with your baby can help in the immediate post-feed period, but your baby spits up right up until the next feed, which means that positioning is only a small part of the fight against reflux.
- *Parents of young babies are tired.* Fighting gravity can be difficult for even the well rested. But take a frustrated, sleep-deprived mother of three and ask her to keep her baby with burning esophagitis vertical for 30 minutes after the 2 A.M. feeding and you've got a recipe for non-compliance. Reality dictates that positioning may be difficult to stay on top of.

But let's keep reality separate from pessimism here. While positioning may not make your baby's reflux simply disappear, it can minimize the exposure of your baby's esophagus and pharynx to irritating acid. For the happy spitter, vertical positioning prevents messes. For the gray-zone baby or the baby with worse reflux, consistent upright positioning will help with sputtering, choking, congestion, and pain. As we'll talk about in the next chapter, one of our goals in treating any baby with reflux is the prevention of injury and complications, and vertical positioning will help with that.

What to Do to Put Gravity on Your Side

- *Keep your baby vertical for 20 to 30 minutes after feeds.* The best way to do this is to rest your baby on your chest so she is looking back over your shoulder. Try as best as possible to keep your baby's body straight up and down. Minimize bending at the hips. The potential downside is that when she burps, it will dribble down your back, but that's what burp cloths are for. Walking or doing chores one-handed is fine and probably a necessary skill for all parents if you haven't mastered it already. The BabyBjörn papoose-style carriers do a wonderful job of helping to maintain vertical positioning and can leave both of your hands free. After age 4 months or so, once a baby is able to maintain head control, hanging bucket-type swings that allow a baby's legs and hips to dangle straight down are helpful in maintaining vertical posture.

- *Avoid aggressive handling.* While terrifying my wife by throwing my daughter high into the air only to catch her on the way down at the very last minute has made for great video footage, it isn't something I did until her reflux was well in check. Avoiding this type of showmanship will help keep the burp cloths clean. Anything that puts pressure on the abdomen, such as holding the baby over your arm or squeezing below the baby's rib cage, will create pressure that influences the forces of reflux. Minimizing extreme changes in position will significantly reduce regurgitation in the refluxing baby.

- *Wedge a baby on her left side.* During the first 2 months of life, babies do a pretty good job of staying where you put them. You can wedge 'em in just about any position and they'll stay. During this period, left-sided positioning with wedges that you can purchase at your local baby store is one of the best ways to keep those acidic gastric contents from that LES, because when the left side is down, stomach contents have a place to pool that's free and clear of the LES.

- *Elevate the head of the crib.* Until your baby begins to move about in her crib, elevation of the head of the crib may help put gravity on your side. Usually 6-inch blocks under the head posts of the crib will create enough elevation to do the trick without making your baby slide. After the first couple of months of life, babies can move to such an extent that this can potentially create a "head down" position that might make matters worse. Another option is to consider investment in a Tucker Sling (www.tuckerdesigns.com). This is a wedge appliance with a Velcro-closure harness that goes right on top of a flat crib mattress. It maintains a 40-degree inclination with gentle restraints that keep your baby put and her head upright.

Despite this advice, the medical research findings on sleep positioning and reflux are mixed as far as whether sleeping at 30 degrees of elevation confers any kind of benefit for the refluxing baby. If you read the medical literature, it may suggest that the effort required to elevate and maintain a child in the head-up position exceeds the benefit. The choice to elevate is a decision you can make on your own, but like many parents, you may be willing to consider anything that can't hurt and might help.

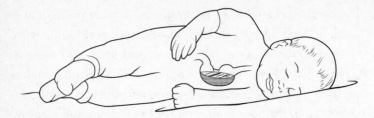

Left-sided positioning during sleep may facilitate the pooling of stomach contents away from the lower esophageal sphincter.

Babies with Reflux Are Like Turtles: A Word About Sleep Position

So after this discussion of positioning, you may be asking yourself, *Do I put my refluxing baby on his belly or back when he's sleeping?* There's a major difference between what may be best for your baby's reflux and what's now considered the recommended sleep position during infancy.

Refluxing babies are like turtles in that they tend to prefer sleeping on their bellies rather than their backs. There's a good reason for this. The LES lies closer to the back of a baby's body, which means that when they're on their backs, milk and tummy acid are more likely to accumulate there and wind up in the esophagus should the LES suddenly relax for a moment. Babies hurting with reflux tend to gravitate away from back positioning once they're able to roll over. For those who can't roll, sleep tends to be sounder belly down.

But as all parents know, babies are supposed to sleep on their backs. It isn't known exactly why, but prone positioning (lying on the belly) has been shown to be associated with SIDS, and efforts to change the way parents put their babies to bed have resulted in fewer SIDS fatalities. So what's a parent with a baby with reflux to do?

There unfortunately isn't a good answer. When the NASPGHAN (North American Society of Pediatric Gastroenterology, Hepatology and Nutrition) tackled the issue of belly versus back for the refluxing baby in its 2001 "Pediatric GE Reflux Clinical Practice Guidelines," it noted that "prone positioning during sleep is only considered in unusual cases where the risk of death from the complications of GER outweighs the potential increased risk of SIDS." They might as well have said: "We know that tummy positioning is associated with SIDS and refluxing babies are sicker on their backs, so look at both options, run the numbers, and choose the lesser of the two evils." Perhaps I'm old-fashioned, but weighing potential methods of death as I wind up my baby's mobile isn't any way to start the evening. But the guidelines' wording reflects the difficult spot that physicians are in when parents ask how they should put their babies down for sleep. Throw in the looming threat of litigation should anything happen to a baby, and you've got a bunch of American physicians fidgeting and tap-dancing their way around the issue.

I've found that, despite physicians' recommendations, position papers, and professional opinions, babies have a way of sorting this out on their own in a way that works for them. I've yet to lose a baby to SIDS or any reflux-related event while sleeping. You should talk to your doctor before settling your baby into any one position. Until then, consider the following options for your baby:

- Irrespective of position, always be sure to use tight, firm bedding on the mattress. No heavy quilts or comforters, please.

- Put the happy spitter and the gray-zone baby to bed on their back. If your baby clearly is in pain and can't sleep, begin with a 30-degree elevation of the head of the bed. Keep in mind, however, that research findings about the effects of head elevation on reflux in babies are mixed.

- If elevation with back positioning doesn't do the trick, consider wedging your baby in a left-side-down position.

- Many babies with reflux esophagitis, especially the bundle of misery and the baby who is sick with reflux, are unable to sleep in any other position than on their tummies. For many parents, the only way to make peace with this option is to keep their baby in their room with them for close supervision. If your baby can sleep only on her tummy and you're unable to keep a close eye on her, consider talking to your doctor about an apnea monitor.

- Some babies sleep on their parents' chest as the parents sit in a recliner. For the short term this is a great way to allow your baby to sleep with real head elevation. But for the long term, this doesn't represent a good solution for you or your baby. You need your rest, and your baby needs to understand that the crib is where she lays her head to sleep. If you're caught in this position, you might look to change.

- And finally, don't believe that allowing baby to sleep next to you in your bed is somehow safer. Crush injuries and asphyxiation have been reported.

Car Seats Are for Car Safety, not Reflux

There's a misconception that car seats represent a great place for the baby with reflux. After all, their heads are higher than the rest of their body, so we've got gravity working for us, right? Not

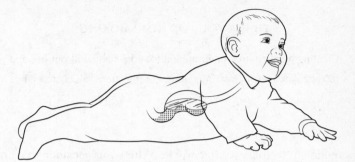

**Prone (belly) positioning often works best
for babies with reflux.**

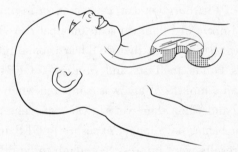

Supine (back) positioning may predispose to reflux.

exactly. Remember that when a baby is on his back, stomach
contents tend to pool near the LES, making reflux more likely
when the baby relaxes his sphincter. Now, if we bend a baby at
the waist and put him bottom down (as in a car seat), we've created a situation in which stomach contents have nowhere to go
but down toward the LES. While your baby does in fact have his
head elevated, his bottom-down position and the distortion of
his anatomy at the junction of the stomach and esophagus have

THANK YOU FOR NOT SMOKING

Creating a smoke-free environment for your baby will put her at a lower risk for respiratory infections, ear infections, SIDS, and GER.

a tendency to make reflux worse. When you consider that infants don't have the ability to sit up during their earlier months, the slumping that naturally occurs increases pressure in the abdominal cavity and contributes to reflux.

Susan Orenstein, M.D., a pediatric gastroenterologist at the University of Pittsburgh and an early pioneer in infant reflux, proved the impact of infant car seats on a baby's reflux. Using pH probes (a test for reflux that we'll learn about in Chapter 8, "A Parent's Guide to Tests and Studies"), GER in babies younger than 6 months of age was compared when they were lying prone and when they were in car seats. The pH probes showed that babies have longer exposure to GER in their car seats. The results were impressive enough to be published in the *New England Journal of Medicine*, a journal that typically doesn't allocate a lot of space to reports about screaming babies.

Let Sleeping Babies Lie

It's important not to be rigid about the reflux care for your bundle of misery. One thing that being a father and pediatrician has taught me is that not all babies read the textbook. Despite our best recommendations, screaming babies sometimes get better with things that just don't seem to make sense. I sometimes encounter babies who seem to be content sleeping only in

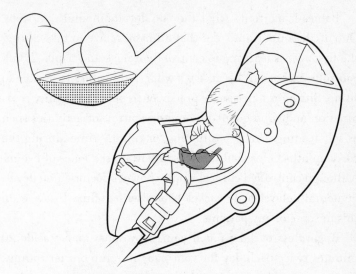

THE ANATOMY OF REFLUX IN A CAR SEAT

The distortion of anatomy while an infant is in a car seat puts her at risk for acid reflux.

a car seat, even though physiology and logic would dictate otherwise. In these situations, it's reasonable to put the *New England Journal of Medicine* on the shelf, trust your judgment, and do what works for you and your baby. All babies are different, as are all babies with reflux. Never mess with what seems to work for your baby.

The Importance of Tummy Time

Some babies spit up so much that their parents don't like to put them down. While I can appreciate the social and hygienic impact of reflux on your household, it's important to understand the role of tummy time in your baby's motor development.

Babies learn to do what they do developmentally in steps. One of the important steps that all babies have to take during the first year is learning to control their neck and trunk. Trunk control is important because it's what helps babies to be able to sit up. Sitting is a necessary precursor to upper extremity coordination and subsequent fine motor control for activities such as self-feeding. Prone positioning, or tummy time, during the early months helps facilitate this important sequence of events. Although controlled clinical studies haven't documented developmental delays in the sicker babies with reflux, I have seen this in some of my patients.

Regardless of how much your baby spits up, set aside 20 minutes twice each day for your baby to romp on her tummy. You can start this after about 1 month of age or as early as when your baby's umbilical cord falls off. A large, soft baby blanket is usually enough to keep the carpets looking fresh.

7

MEDICATIONS FOR REFLUX

To Treat or Not to Treat?

Several years before Donald Trump's meteoric rise to fame, he was pictured on the cover of one of the grocery store tabloids holding his screaming baby Tiffany. With a sour grimace caught at just the right moment, the picture and the headline tell everything of the Donald's life with a baby "that won't stop crying." While the clinical details of Tiffany's health were missing, it was reported that the family sought chiropractic treatment for her as a means of getting relief. This demonstrates that the impact of a baby's misery knows no boundaries of privilege and that parents will even submit their babies to spinal manipulation to get relief.

Desperation is a feeling experienced by many parents of babies with acid reflux. And aromatherapy and chiropractic are just a couple of the extreme measures that parents will resort to when faced with the feeling that there's nothing that can help their baby. In many cases, desperation is unnecessary—the parents are under the misperception that nothing can be done, which is sometimes perpetuated by physicians who tell the parents that because their baby's gaining weight, there's nothing to worry about. But today's pediatricians have at their disposal new therapies for treating the baby with intractable irritability due to reflux.

JUST WHAT ARE WE TRYING TO ACHIEVE?

What are physicians trying to achieve in the baby with reflux? Well, according to the treatment guidelines set forth by NASPGHAN, our goals of treating reflux should be the following:

- Relieve symptoms
- Promote normal weight gain
- Heal inflammation
- Prevent complications

Or, more simply put, we want them to feel better, grow, and not get any worse. For the bundle of misery, this equates to less screaming and "colicky" behavior. For the gray-zone baby, it could mean feeding easier and more efficiently with less fussing. This sounds like a reasonable set of goals, but the devil's in the details. Which babies do we treat?

TO TREAT OR NOT TO TREAT—THAT IS THE QUESTION

One of the great difficulties in treating reflux is the subjective experience of the individual looking at the baby. One parent's spit-up is another parent's crisis. Excessive screaming to one person is a minor deviation in temperament; to another it's a sign of a problem that must be addressed. For a baby's symptoms, pain is in the eye of the beholder, or, more precisely, the holder.

This contrast is played out every day in pediatricians' offices. Take, for example, the physician who, during a 7-minute office visit, finds a sleeping baby with good weight gain and a report from the family that the baby is miserable. The doctor may have the impression of a perfectly normal baby with anxious, first-time parents. For the parents who must live with the baby for the remaining 23 hours and 53 minutes of that day, the impression of their baby—who screams, arches, can't sleep, and can't feed—will be quite different. Depending on how the visit plays out, this child will either be treated for symptoms of acid reflux or sent home with gas drops and a clean bill of health.

Because of all the variables, the decision to treat is unfortunately often based on the time and effort put forth by the physician to elicit the subtle symptoms of reflux as well as the parents' ability to assertively detail their baby's experience. If any of these parties charged with advocating for the baby's health fails to do what he or she should be doing, the result is untreated symptoms and frustration.

As we've discussed at some length, there are different degrees of acid reflux. The sick babies should be easily identified by a thorough pediatrician. The happy spitters similarly can be identified through a physician's persistent inquiry. It's the many gray-zone babies who create the real dilemma. They can look good but live in pain, creating a real problem for family dynamics. And though everyone agrees that the happy spitter almost never needs therapy and that the baby sick with reflux always needs therapy, we may never be able to get two physicians to agree on the kids in between.

I think that most reasonable-minded pediatricians, when faced with reasonable-minded parents who describe feeding difficulty, marked sleep disturbance, and marked irritability consistent with reflux, would agree to a trial of treatment for a baby. If you don't have a reasonable-minded pediatrician, you've got a different issue on your hands. In Chapter 9, "What to Expect from Your Physician," we'll discuss how best to handle the situation of a physician who won't listen or take the time to understand your baby's symptoms. For now, let's discuss the options available for treating your baby with reflux.

THE MEDICAL APPROACH TO THE CHILD WITH REFLUX

The medical approach to treating reflux in babies is pretty straightforward. It involves addressing the issue of *stomach acid*, which creates the pain of reflux, and *stomach emptying*, which is one of the key initiators of reflux. If we can get these two problems in line, you're likely to see a happier baby who feeds and sleeps better.

Acid Suppression

Stomach acid is the trigger that makes refluxing babies scream. If we can decrease the amount of acid that your baby's esophagus encounters, you should have a happier baby. This is what acid suppressants do; they decrease exposure of the esophagus to acid by cutting the amount of acid that's produced by the stomach. When the esophagus heals and becomes happier, it's better able to let food and milk through and babies can then feed more peacefully. The effects of acid blockade go beyond feeding, of course. Many of those signs and symptoms involv-

WHY YOUR BABY DOESN'T GET BETTER AFTER TAKING GAS DROPS

You may be seduced into buying "gas drops" for your screaming baby. What are these, and what do they do? Based on the idea that colic is due to gas, these over-the-counter preparations help break up gas. Most contain simethicone, a compound that does a pretty good job of making big gas bubbles into small ones. You've gone half bankrupt on gas drops, but still he screams, cries, and farts like a frat boy. Why is this?

- *Really big gas is his problem.* While simethicone does a reasonably good job of breaking down gas bubbles, the problem is that the volume of gas taken in by the baby with reflux, or any screaming baby for that matter, is too great to be dealt with by a few drops of simethicone.
- *Babies do not scream from gas alone.* Remember that despite swallowing air and having gas, babies don't scream because of gas alone. Other factors such as reflux esophagitis, milk protein allergy, and temperament are in play.

But hope springs eternal, and as long as there are desperate parents with babies carrying the diagnosis of colic, there will be gas drops.

ing the throat and breathing that we talked about in Chapters 3 and 4 will decrease when acid exposure is diminished.

Physicians can use two classes of medication to suppress acid in babies: *histamine₂-receptor antagonists* (*H₂RAs*) and *proton pump inhibitors* (*PPIs*). The degree of your baby's symptoms and your physician's level of comfort with various

medications will determine which of these two types of medication will be a fundamental part of your baby's treatment.
Both types work by decreasing the acid that's produced by the
stomach.

Histamine$_2$-Receptor Antagonists

Known to most of us as Zantac, Axid, and Pepcid, H$_2$RAs have
been with us for some time, at least since 1981. Physicians are
familiar with the performance and track record of these drugs,
especially because for the longest time, they were the only
treatment that we knew of for acid-related symptoms in children.

The name comes from the type of cell receptor, or switch,
that sits at the base of the stomach's acid-producing cells.
When triggered, or switched on by the chemical histamine, the
parietal cells are stimulated to make acid. Our bodies do this
under normal circumstances or in situations in which we may
need extra acid, such as when eating. H$_2$-receptor *antagonists*
block the triggering of this cell switch and in turn decrease the
amount of acid produced by the parietal cells. Unfortunately,
there are other triggers and switches that will stimulate acid
production in parietal cells, so blocking the H$_2$ receptor in the
stomach isn't enough to fix every acid-related problem. Because H$_2$RAs have been available for a long time, physicians are
confident about their use. Their safety profile is excellent and
their side effects are minimal, two factors of major importance
when choosing the therapy that's prescribed.

For the baby with mild symptoms of reflux esophagitis,
H$_2$RAs represent a reasonable treatment option. But one of the
major problems with this class of acid blockers is that they tend

to lose their effectiveness with time. For reasons that are unclear, individuals undergoing long-term treatment have been reported to have breakthroughs in their symptoms as early as 6 weeks into treatment, a phenomenon referred to as *tachyphylaxis*. This has also been observed in infants.

Proton Pump Inhibitors

Though H2RAs block one of several switches that turn on the acid pumps in the stomach, why not go directly to the source and block the pumps altogether? That's possible through the use of PPIs, which work to stop the release of acid at the tip of the parietal cells where it's released into the stomach. As you can imagine, stopping the pumps that release the acid is one of the most effective ways to control acid production.

Stopping acid production at its source sounds like the way to go. PPIs do a better job at controlling acid-related diseases than other medications such as H2RAs. Numerous studies in adults have shown that PPIs are superior to H2RAs at blocking acid secretion and healing the damaged esophagus. The healing rates in children with esophagitis are higher with PPIs than with H2RAs.

Proton Pump Inhibitors in Kids: Is There a Track Record?

The issue of safety with medications in children is often an issue because the pharmaceutical world is centered around adults. After all, adulthood is when bodies start falling apart, and it's the chronic diseases of adulthood that require the medications that drive profits and keep the pharmaceutical industry innovative. Because the numbers aren't there to financially justify bringing new drugs to the marketplace just for children,

HOW DO YOU DIGEST FOOD IF YOU
DON'T HAVE STOMACH ACID?

Acid blockers don't completely eliminate digestive juices in the stomach. There's plenty of acid available for the stomach to do its job, which is to break down foods to their more basic elements for digestion in the intestine.

testing for children often occurs after safety and effectiveness have been proven in adults. As inequitable as it may sound, it's the way our system works.

Because of this, pediatricians have a tendency to see what's new in adults and then try it out in children. But don't get the wrong idea. It's not that we experiment when it comes to kids; it's just that sometimes the clinical studies lag behind the actual use of a medication. There are exceptions, but medications with good track records in adults tend to have good track records in children.

This is the case with PPIs, which first came into use in the adult population in 1989 with the U.S. Food and Drug Administration (FDA) approval of Prilosec (omeprazole). Its amazing ability to squelch stomach acid and heal ulcers led to its being touted as a miracle drug. At the time, there were concerns that chronic suppression of stomach acid could lead to stomach cancer, but later studies in adults who had been treated continuously with PPIs for several years failed to show any connection with cancer.

While not initially approved for use in young children, omeprazole was popularly prescribed by pediatric gastroenterologists starting in the mid-1990s. At the time, it was thought that the benefit derived by children with reflux disease from PPIs outweighed the potential risks. And as time passed, physicians became more comfortable with the belief that PPIs represented a safe, effective therapy for adults and children alike.

At the time, there were some curious pediatric gastroenterologists who thought that PPIs might be worth a shot in miserable babies. Information was becoming more available that many babies suffering with intractable coliclike symptoms actually had acid reflux. The results reported by some clinicians early on were remarkable; babies who had been referred for symptoms of severe reflux esophagitis that hadn't responded to traditional therapy seemed to get better. This was my own experience as I began treating babies with PPIs in the mid-1990s. As I began treating more and more screaming babies labeled with colic, I was sold on the medication's effectiveness and quickly earned a reputation among referring pediatricians as someone with insight into a problem that had been plaguing them for decades.

The Food and Drug Administration Approves Proton Pump Inhibitor Use in Children

As PPIs took hold as a mainstay of therapy in children with acid-related disorders, their prescription became more widespread among pediatric gastroenterologists. In 2002 the FDA approved the use of Prevacid (lansoprazole) in children older than 12 months of age. In 2006 the FDA approved the use of Nexium (esomeprazole) in children over the age of 11 years. Clinical studies examining their safety has showed little in the way of concerning side effects, and this has been borne out in my treatment of thousands of children over the past several years.

So what about babies? If the FDA has approved the use of selected PPIs in children, can we feel comfortable with their use in children younger than 1 year of age? The best answer is that there isn't any evidence to suggest that it's a problem. Remember that many of the drugs that we currently use in children are not formally approved by the FDA because the trials necessary to make the federal government satisfied with their unequivocal safety haven't yet been conducted. But as I mentioned earlier, PPIs have been in use in babies since the mid-1990s, and so far there has been nothing to suggest a problem.

Beyond what even the best clinical studies can show, there's nothing about a child's digestive system to suggest that PPIs work in a way that's much different from how they work in an adult. Preliminary results of a clinical study released in 2005 looking at the effects of long-term PPI use (an average of 3 years) in children as young as 6 months of age showed little in the way of effects on stomach physiology. The authors of the study did conclude their report by suggesting that their findings be backed up with longer-term studies in children.

So while everyone agrees that there's work to be done as far as studying babies who take PPIs, the drugs have an excellent track record, they've been prescribed by pediatric gastroenterologists for more than a decade, and the risk-to-benefit balance makes them seem a reasonable option for babies suffering with reflux. The very subjective issue of risk versus benefit becomes important when getting help for your baby because some physicians who have little experience with the latest therapeutic options for screaming babies may not be able to weigh the risks appropriately. In other words, if your pediatrician's never prescribed PPIs to treat reflux, she's unlikely to start now, no matter how miserable your baby may be (more on this in Chapter 9, "What to Expect from Your Physician").

Prokinetic Therapy: Is Cutting Acid Enough?

The Why of Prokinetics

GER in babies is usually a temporary issue that arises from intestinal physiology that isn't quite up to speed. And while using antacids tends to work for many of the most irritating symptoms, sometimes it may not be enough. Improving a child's intestinal motility is another option, so your physician may choose to use a medication referred to as a *prokinetic* medication. For those of you rusty on your Greek, this originates from the Greek term that means "to move." Prokinetic medications can have a variety of effects on intestinal movement that may affect a baby's reflux:

- Increased esophageal squeezing
- Increased LES pressure
- Accelerated stomach emptying

The problem is that the results of studies looking at the effectiveness of these medications in improving reflux are contradictory. Some studies show an effect; others seem to find them almost worthless. Interestingly, this mirrors what physicians find clinically: Some babies have a brilliant response to prokinetics, whereas others have a very lackluster response. This leads me to **Reflux rule 4: Treating reflux is a lot like shopping for shoes—you never know what's going to work until you try it on.** This is especially true when it comes to prokinetics. Just as the clinical studies bear out, the response to them is mixed.

Why is this—why don't babies' bodies respond predictably? It probably relates to what we discussed back in Chapter 2 ("Reflux 101"): that reflux most likely represents more than one condition. A variety of physiologic issues related to motility can occur, from frequent LES relaxations to poor tummy emptying, exactly which issue predominates in any one baby is practically impossible to determine. Even though most pediatric gastroenterologists would agree that the response to prokinetic agents is iffy, most would also agree that they're definitely worth a try in the baby with problem reflux. As with a fine pair of Ferragamo pumps, you've got to try them on to know if they'll work for you.

Reglan and Bethanechol, Potential Prokinetics

If your physician chooses to use a prokinetic, it will most likely be either Reglan (metoclopramide) or Urecholine (bethanechol). A friendly piece of advice: Don't pick an argument about the conflicting medical literature. Just assume your physician is on the side of those who have had pretty good luck with the drug over the years. Here are a few things you should know about these medications that may not be discussed at your visit:

- *Timing isn't everything.* Both medications are given three to four times per day. Technically, you should be timing these medications 30 minutes before feeding your baby, but often the reality of the situation prevents this. If you can't time it right, don't keep your baby screaming for a half hour. Go ahead and give the dose and give the feeding a little early if necessary. If you wait the half hour, the air and gas that she takes in protesting will counter any effect seen from the medication. It isn't dangerous to fudge the timing; it's just that the effect may not be entirely optimal. I like to tell families that if they can get two of the four daily doses timed 30 minutes before a feeding, they're doing a great job.

Along these lines, parents are often told that the medication must be given about every 6 hours. If you stick strictly to this, the odds of dosing your baby 30 minutes before a feeding at the 6-hour mark with her not being asleep are virtually impossible. I tell families to administer three of the prokinetic doses during "waking hours" as close as 4 hours apart if necessary to get the timing right. If you can work the fourth dose in in the middle of the night, great. Otherwise, that fourth dose may not make a lot of difference as far as your child's symptoms.

· *You might need to find a compounding pharmacy.* Metoclopramide is available as a prepared liquid; bethanechol has to be compounded, or mixed into a liquid, by a pharmacist. Many of the chain pharmacies don't provide this service, so ask your physician or call ahead before wasting a trip to the pharmacy.

· *Changes in baby's behavior.* Metoclopramide has been associated with sleepiness, sleeplessness, jittery behavior, and a rare complication referred to as tardive dyskinesia. Babies with tardive dyskinesia commonly engage in extreme arching, head turning, and tongue thrusting. This typically goes away with a little diphenhydramine (Benadryl) and discontinuation of the metoclopramide. With the exception of the side effects seen with metoclopramide, both medications have been around for a long time and have reasonably good safety records. Any unusual changes seen in your baby when starting a prokinetic, or any medication for that matter, should prompt an immediate call to your physician.

- *Prokinetics, medications best served cold.* While metoclopramide may be stored at room temperature, bethanechol may require refrigeration depending upon how it's prepared. Because compounds can vary, be sure to discuss temperature requirements with your pharmacist.

TO TREAT OR NOT TO TREAT—PULLING OUR OPTIONS TOGETHER

We've talked about different antacids and controversial motility medications for your baby. What should you expect when seeking treatment for your baby? That depends on your baby and your physician. Remember that sick babies are almost always treated, happy spitters are almost never treated, and gray-zone babies are in the eye of the beholder . . . or holder. Remember that how your physician sees your gray-zone baby may depend on how familiar he is with reflux and how comfortable he is with your baby's story. But despite how well you relate your baby's symptoms or how young your pediatrician may be, any of the following signs and symptoms due to reflux in your baby may be indications for therapy:

- Difficulty feeding
- Marked irritability
- Failure to gain weight appropriately
- Airway symptoms, including congestion, choking, and chronic cough

PROPULCID: THE CAUTIONARY TALE OF A MIRACLE PROKINETIC GONE BAD

When the U.S. stock market went hog wild in the late 1990s, some-one wrote a book called *Irrational Exuberance*. It described the fi-nancial feeding frenzy of that decade that drove everyone to think that the market was going to go up forever. And we all know how that turned out. The book's title and story reminds me of a similar frenzy among physicians that occurred in the same period about a medication called Propulcid (cisapride). Propulcid was a remark-ably effective prokinetic medication that was approved for the treat-ment of reflux. Its ability to conquer the worst reflux made Propulcid the new darling of the pediatric gastroenterology com-munity. Propulcid was even evolving as a miracle drug in the treat-ment of a variety of bowel motility disorders in adults.

But all wasn't as it seemed. Reports began appearing of a subtle change in the heart rhythm of patients treated with Propulcid. More specifically, some patients treated with it had a very slight prolon-gation of the heart's electrical "recovery," seen on an electrocardio-gram. For most patients, this wasn't a problem. But for those with an uncommon rhythm disturbance known as *prolonged QT syndrome*, Propulcid had the ability to send their heart into a fatal electrical pattern. Several sudden deaths occurred, mostly among adults with frail hearts. The manufacturer was forced to remove Propulcid from the U.S. market. Though it is a phenomenal drug, its overnight suc-cess and indiscriminate overuse were ultimately responsible for its demise.

Pediatricians remember that brief interlude with the medication that brought so many kids relief but had the potential for life-threatening problems in a few. As a consequence, many primary

care physicians now make it a policy to refer children needing specialty medications to specialists such as pediatric gastroenterologists. The Propulcid story has taught us that regardless of how
miraculous a new medication's effect may be, no drug is risk free
and treatment decisions always must be made with utmost caution.

So what can you expect to happen that will get your baby feeling better?

Acid Suppression Therapy Is Often Enough

Acid suppression is enough to make many babies feel better,
which should be the minimum. In many respects, this represents a good option because it involves only one medication.
And with acid suppressants, side effects are minimal.

But reflux is a motility disorder. Will acid suppressants
make reflux go away? Not necessarily, but they will often
make conditions a lot more tolerable. There are a number of
ways that acid suppression alone can conceivably make your
baby's reflux better: Remember that it's the irritation of the
esophagus and throat that creates the painful burning sensation that babies experience while feeding. And remember that an irritated esophagus strips, or clears, reflux acid
less efficiently, so relieving that inflammation allows a baby's
body to protect itself better. Gastric irritation from excessive acid production or allergic reactivity is likely to decrease with acid suppression, making tummy emptying more
efficient.

Histamine$_2$-Receptor Antagonist or Proton Pump Inhibitor?

For mild reflux, an H$_2$RA may be enough to conquer your baby's irritability from painful reflux. Administration of an H$_2$RA may be difficult, depending on how your physician chooses to prescribe it. In one of its most commonly prescribed forms for babies, liquid Zantac (ranitidine) is prepared in an alcohol-based solution that has a very strong menthol taste. Some babies take it without a hitch, but I've seen many gag and scream over its noxious taste. Some argue that alcohol-based liquid medications shouldn't be used in babies, but the amount probably isn't enough to get excited about if your baby tolerates it. Zantac is also available in an EFFERdose packet that can be suspended in water and given to a baby.

Though ranitidine may provide adequate relief for some babies, I am biased toward the use of PPIs, which more effectively treat acid problems in both adults and children. The dosing of PPIs, which are given only once or twice a day, is an advantage over that for H$_2$RAs, which are given as many as three times a day. And don't forget the fact that H$_2$RAs have a tendency to lose their effectiveness after a couple of months of use.

I don't mean to knock H$_2$RAs, but I prescribe them infrequently. As someone who deals with children referred for difficult-to-manage reflux, I favor the most definitive therapy. But for a baby who doesn't seem remarkably sick and who's being treated by a family practitioner or pediatrician, H$_2$RAs may be a reasonable place to start.

Some physicians decide to treat with an H$_2$RA not because it represents the best treatment for a baby but because they have reservations about other forms of acid suppression such as

PPIs. Old habits die hard, and some physicians are more comfortable seeing a class of medication pass the test of time before prescribing it for their patients. H_2RAs may not be quite as effective as calming babies with reflux esophagitis, but I always tell pediatricians that it's better to treat babies with something than to leave them in pain.

Step Up Versus Step Down

Your pediatrician may recommend that your baby have it both ways through a step-up or step-down approach. This approach to treating reflux takes advantage of the healing power of PPIs with the reasonable effectiveness of H_2RAs at keeping symptoms under control. In the step-down approach, babies or children are first given a PPI for, say, a couple of months to get things under control and are then given an H_2RA for the long haul. This plan addresses the theoretical concern of prolonged PPI use while keeping costs under control.

The step-up approach is to begin first with an H_2RA to try to achieve control of symptoms and then advance to a PPI should the H_2RA not work. The step-up approach is a very reasonable approach to the baby with reflux, although it depends on the baby's symptoms. From my personal experience as well as from having worked with hundreds of other parents with irritable babies, I know that Mom and Dad tend to be short on patience when it comes to a baby who can't feed and can't sleep.

Picking Potential Proton Pump Inhibitors

If your physician chooses to treat your child with a PPI, she has some options. As a general rule, however, there isn't a lot of dif-

PROTON PUMP INHIBITORS—BETTER BUT NOT NECESSARILY STRONGER

Keep in mind that a more effective medication doesn't necessarily mean a stronger medication. PPIs simply work better at tackling the symptoms of acid reflux in both adults and babies. There's no evidence that there's anything more strong or powerful about PPIs; they just work in a more efficient way.

ference among the different PPIs when it comes to effectiveness in treating acid-related problems in children. There are few studies showing head-to-head comparison of these medications when treating kids. In adults, who often have more advanced damage in the esophagus, there are studies showing greater effectiveness of one medication over another in different situations. Children tend not to have the kind of advanced damage that can be followed, measured, and compared so easily. But for reasons that aren't entirely clear, some children will do better with one PPI than another. This, of course, supports my fourth reflux rule, which states that treating reflux is a lot like buying shoes. Not all size 5½ shoes feel the same.

As we've discussed previously, even though the FDA has approved the use of some PPIs in children as young as 12 months of age, they're commonly prescribed by pediatric gastroenterologists for infants with significant reflux symptoms. Prilosec is approved for use in children 2 years of age and older and has the advantage of having been used for more than a decade in infants with significant acid reflux.

Omeprazole might seem like the most logical choice, given

the fact that it was the first PPI approved back in the 1980s, but managed care has created a few hang-ups. The problem begins with the fact that omeprazole is available for over-the-counter use. So when prescriptions are written for it, the insurance companies immediately reject coverage because they believe that policy holders can simply run to the neighborhood drugstore and buy it. But the omeprazole that is currently available over the counter cannot be opened and administered to a baby in the way that other PPIs can. *Easy enough*, you think. *We'll just explain this to the nice person at the other end of the 1-800 customer-service number.* Good luck. PPIs are expensive, and insurance companies are doing everything they can to control their prescription costs. Expect some resistance.

Baby-Friendly Forms of Protein Pump Inhibitors

Assuming that you don't have an administrative staff of your own to generate the barrage of phone calls and endless letters necessary to get your insurance company to cover omeprazole, your doctor may consider an alternative choice of PPI. Lansoprazole (Prevacid) is the most commonly used PPI in children, and it's available in two forms that are easy to administer:

- *Orally disintegrating tablet:* Designed for easy administration to pill-fearing children, the orally disintegrating tablet can easily be administered to babies. A dose of approximately 7.5 milligrams can be delivered by breaking a 15-milligram tablet in two and dissolving half of the tablet in a teaspoon of water. The tablet dissolves in a matter of seconds and can then be given to your baby directly with a small spoon or drawn up into a syringe and admin-

COMMON ACID SUPPRESSANTS USED FOR GASTROESOPHAGEAL REFLUX DISEASE IN INFANCY

Brand Name	Generic Name	FDA Approval for Age	Available Form	Commonly Used Dose*	Note
Zantac	Ranitidine	1 month–16 years	Liquid EFFERdose tablet	5–10 mg/kg per day in 2–3 divided doses	Alcohol base of liquid form is repulsive
Axid	Nizatidine	Older than 12 years	Capsule Oral solution	2.5 mg/kg twice daily	Supposed to taste like bubble gum
Prilosec	Omeprazole	Older than 24 months	Capsule	5 mg once or twice daily	Omeprazole does not have FDA approval for use in infancy. Over-the-counter omeprazole cannot be opened and sprinkled in food.
Prevacid	Lansoprazole	Older than 12 months	Orally dis-integrating tablet Capsule Powder pack	7.5 mg once or twice daily	Lansoprazole does not have FDA approval for use in infancy but is commonly used

* Medication dosing of acid suppressants is based on a baby's size and severity of symptoms. Talk to your physician for the dose that's appropriate for your child. While the information has been left out here for simplicity, some of the above medications are available in intravenous form.

FDA = Food and Drug Administration
kg = kilogram
mg = milligram

istered that way. Another option that has worked for some parents is to put half of the tablet on the tip of their finger and place it into the baby's cheek. Keep your finger on the tab, and you'll feel it disintegrate in a matter of several seconds. Follow up with a bottle or pacifier. Don't dissolve the tablet in your baby's bottle—some of the medication may stick to the bottle or in the nipple. And if she doesn't finish her bottle, she's at risk of not getting her medicine.

- *Capsule:* An alternative to the orally disintegrating tablet is to open up a capsule and administer the tiny beads that are inside. A dose of approximately 7.5 milligrams can be delivered by first opening up a 15-milligram capsule and emptying half of the beads onto a smooth countertop or small bowl. Keep the second half of the capsule in a safe place if your baby is prescribed a second dose for that day. Moisten your finger with breast milk or formula and touch the beads. They will stick to your finger. Then sweep your finger into your baby's cheek and follow up with a pacifier, breast, or bottle. These beads are small enough to be swallowed by babies without any difficulty. And don't worry if a few wind up coming out. The beads can also be mixed in with a small amount of applesauce if your baby is already eating solids or if your pediatrician says it's okay.

    If you can get omeprazole prescribed, it too can be given this way. Keep in mind that the number of milligrams in an omeprazole capsule is different than in a lansoprazole capsule. This doesn't mean that one is stronger than the other; it's just the way the medications are manufactured. Talk to your physician about appropriate dosing in your baby.

    Whatever you do, resist the temptation to smash these beads into a pulp. You may think that doing so will make it easier for your baby to take the medication, but you may be making the medication less effective. PPIs are quite sensitive and lose their effectiveness when exposed to the acid environment of the stomach, so when they are manufactured, the active drug is nestled comfortably in the center of these little beads that protect the medication and allow it to be released slowly and safely.

But My Pharmacist Says She Can Put This into a Suspension

Another option that your doctor or pharmacist may suggest is that your baby's PPI be made into a liquid suspension. What happens in this case is the PPI beads are crushed and put into a suspension along with neutralizing bicarbonate, which is supposed to help counter the effect of stomach acid and keep the drug safe and active. But these medications don't tolerate the harsh environment of medicine bottles, and the effects of direct exposure in the stomach without their protective beads make this not the best option. Having seen hundreds of children who initially took compounded PPI suspensions improve when switched to an intact form of the medicine, I feel that the effectiveness of PPIs is diminished when manipulated for syrupy suspension.

What to Expect from Treatment

So you've convinced your physician to abandon the catch-all diagnosis of colic and believe that your screaming, spitting, congested, hiccupping, sleepless, difficult-to-feed baby needs a little help. Your baby has begun therapy. Now what should you expect? When should your baby feel better?

For the most miserable babies with reflux, initiation of ther-

THE MOM WHO COUNTED EVERY BEAD

Once, the mother of one of my patients took my advice of a "half capsule twice daily" quite literally. She would start her day by opening her child's PPI capsule to count the number of beads enclosed. She then distributed the beads into two piles for precise administration. When she brought her baby in for a follow-up visit 4 weeks later, she proudly reported her daily diligence. I was tempted to suggest that she needed to get out of the house more, but I held my tongue, realizing that this was just an extreme expression of a mother's love. Given the safety of PPIs, it's believed that there is a fairly wide range of doses that can comfortably be used. When splitting a capsule, it's reasonable to eyeball the dose with the understanding that a tiny bit less this morning means a tiny bit more this evening.

apy with a PPI will result in some improvement within 3 to 5 days. For many, however, pain relief may take longer. Clinical studies show that maximum improvement may not be seen for 4 weeks, although it's the exceptional baby who shows no improvement until 4 weeks into treatment. If after 2 to 3 weeks your baby is just as miserable as the day treatment began, it may be time to consider alternate causes of your baby's misery or changes in her reflux regimen. Signs of improvement include

- Improved sleep quality
- Less irritability, crying, and fussiness
- More comfortable, effortless feeding
- Less gas

SPITTIN' PURPLE

The material inside the timed-release beads of some of the PPIs contain a bluish purple tint that looks almost like squished blueberries. You may occasionally see streaks of this on the burp cloth; it's nothing to worry about. However, if the material looks brown or black, like coffee grounds, you should notify your doctor immediately, because this could be blood.

Adding a Prokinetic for Good Measure

One option that can be considered in the baby whose reflux doesn't respond to acid suppression alone is the addition of a prokinetic. As we've discussed, their effectiveness in turning sick babies around is unequivocal, although physicians who frequently treat reflux in children have had enough success with prokinetics to make their use a viable consideration. Some physicians will initially treat with both a prokinetic and an acid suppressant as a means of trying to achieve the best effect by the quickest means possible. Prokinetics and acid suppressants can be comfortably used together.

Treating Reflux Is a Lot Like Steering a Boat

Parents of miserable babies tend to be impatient. They want results yesterday. But as we've learned, acid-suppression therapy often works quickly—but that may translate to 2 to 4 weeks. When they work, prokinetics tend to show results quicker, as far as decreasing spitting up and improving gastric

ERYTHROMYCIN—AN ANTIBIOTIC FOR REFLUX?

Your pediatric gastroenterologist may recommend erythromycin for your baby's reflux. How crazy is that? Is it time to find a new physician? Not necessarily. Erythromycin stimulates a switch on intestinal muscle cells that initiates motility. Because of this convenient little pharmacologic quirk, erythromycin is sometimes used in difficult-to-treat cases of reflux when other prokinetics haven't worked. The results are mixed, but it may be worth a try.

emptying. But even with prokinetics, you may need to be patient for 1 to 2 weeks before considering them helpful or not. The bottom line is that once you and your physician take an approach to treatment, you need to hang in there. That leads me to **Reflux rule 5: Treating reflux is a lot like steering a sailboat—changing direction takes time.** If you've ever had the opportunity to steer a sailboat, you know that unlike the way things work with a car, if you want to change direction you need to plot your course, change tack, and wait for the boat to come around. Quickly pulling back and forth on the rudder does nothing. And so it goes for the baby with reflux symptoms. Therapies take time to have an effect. A badly irritated esophagus doesn't get better overnight. So no matter what treatment your doctor recommends, be patient and hang in there.

Quickly jumping on and off medications because of unreasonable expectations will always create more frustration than relief. Sometimes you have to take the advice of one of my sage medical school professors, who impressed on students the criti-

> ## WHAT TO DO WHEN THE BABY WHO SPITS UP ALL THE TIME SPITS UP THE MEDICINE INTENDED TO HELP HIS SPITTING UP
>
> If your baby spits up his medication, it's safe in most cases to repeat the dose of medication if it is spit up within 15 to 20 minutes of administration. It's rare that an infant spits up so much that he can't keep down so much as a dose of medication.

cal importance of patience by saying, "Don't just do something—stand there."

A Word About Antacids and Things That Coat the Throat

Okay, it's 2 A.M. and you're awakened from a dead sleep by a piercing scream coming from the nursery. You stumble out of bed to find your baby arching, gulping, and grimacing. You pick her up, and she settles down a bit, but she's clearly in pain, writhing and turning her head. Acid-suppression therapy was started just 2 days earlier and you know it's too early to expect much of an effect. What can you do?

One option is to do for your baby what you might do for yourself, and that is to reach for a bottle of Mylanta or Maalox. Offer about half a teaspoon (2 to 3 milliliters) of one of these topical antacids, and you may be able to buy 20 minutes of relief. This helps when babies are suffering with throat and esophagus pain from their reflux.

As a general rule, this isn't something that you should make a habit of, but once every day or two until your baby's acid suppressant kicks in shouldn't be a problem. Be sure to talk to your physician first, because this can be dangerous for babies with certain problems such as kidney disease.

Your physician may prescribe a small dose of Carafate (sucralfate) for temporary use. Carafate doesn't neutralize acid, it sticks to the inflamed, eroded intestinal lining. It's most frequently used in adults with stomach ulcers to help with healing. Your baby most likely doesn't have an eroded esophagus lining, but Carafate can offer relief in some babies. Like antacids, it's not for long-term use and can be prescribed only for healthy babies.

KNOWING WHEN TO LET GO: HOW DO YOU KNOW WHEN TO STOP A BABY'S REFLUX MEDICATION?

Once your baby gets to feeling and feeding better, you may be tempted to never risk anything that could ever have your baby feeling bad again, such as discontinuing her medications. But the day will come when they're not needed. Despite how bad things may seem early on, we know that most cases of reflux in babies resolve on their own. When a baby is between 4 and 12 months of age, his capacity to empty his tummy and keep things out of his esophagus generally improves. As this happens, you might tend to attribute your happy, healthy baby's bliss to his medications and not to natural changes in his physiology. Medications can become good-luck charms that we always want to have with us.

How will you know when your baby is ready to stop taking his medications? The honest truth is that there typically aren't flags that point the way for you and your physician. In many cases, physicians take a leap of faith, knowing what they know about babies and reflux. Here are some signs that your baby may *not* be ready to stop taking medications:

- Your baby continues to have bothersome reflux symptoms.
- Missed doses lead to reflux symptoms.
- Your baby has other symptoms, such as feeding difficulty or lung problems, despite no longer having ongoing reflux symptoms.

Assuming that your baby has made a brilliant recovery and has little in the way of reflux symptoms, it may be reasonable to consider stopping medications. In some babies with mild symptoms that have decreased, it may be reasonable to consider this as early as 8 weeks after medications were begun. In the sicker baby, the bundle of misery, or the baby whose symptoms were more difficult to get under control, it's often wiser to push them further along toward 8 to 10 months of age before removing medical support. This decision must be made between you and your physician and will depend on your child's medical history and his current clinical status. Every child is different, but medications are almost never forever.

The way medications are discontinued will vary from physician to physician. In a baby being treated with a prokinetic and an antacid, I usually first discontinue the prokinetic to see how things go. If all's well in, say, 2 to 3 weeks, I will discontinue the acid suppression. I usually instruct parents that if they notice any regression in symptoms at any point, they should revert to the last level of therapy. And sometimes we lose perspective when treating reflux. Remember that reflux in infancy is a normal, physiologic process. If a little increase in spitting up is noted with removal of medication, I encourage parents to ride it out.

As a general rule, I prefer to discontinue medications cold turkey when I think that a baby is ready. The reason is that this better allows me to see a black-and-white difference in the baby's feeding and behavior than if I were to wean or taper the medications as some physicians recommend. The times when I've tapered reflux medications in infancy, there's often been some other speed bump such as teething or upper respiratory infections that appear just as we're trying to make decisions about reflux symptoms.

WHAT TO CONSIDER WHEN BABY DOESN'T GET BETTER

What if your baby with reflux has been treated but she doesn't get better? When this occurs, you should ask your doctor a few questions:

- *Have medications been maximized?* Many medications are prescribed on the basis of the baby's weight and there is a range of potential doses available. Sometimes children have to be treated on the higher end of the dose range before there is a change.
- *Have we given our treatments enough time?* Remember that the changes that come with treatment sometimes take a couple of weeks or longer. Don't throw in the burp cloth too early.
- *Is there anything else wrong with my baby?* Remember that all that spits isn't reflux. Though they're less often the culprit, a variety of problems can lead to vomiting and

screaming in babies. Your pediatrician or pediatric gastroenterologist should help you understand what's to be expected in the baby with reflux.

- *Do you have enough heads on the case?* Sometimes two heads are better than one. If your baby isn't responding in a way you or your pediatrician expects, you might ask about a referral to a pediatric gastroenterologist. This kind of specialist is best able to judge whether your baby has reached the end of her rope as far as medications are concerned.

KNOWING WHEN TO THROW IN THE BURP CLOTH

Despite our best efforts, your baby simply may not be the happiest baby on the block. Bona fide reflux doesn't always respond to the medications that we have in the way that we would expect. For parents who live in a world of immediate gratification, it's a stark reality.

When this happens, we have to take a look at our babies and sometimes ourselves. We first have to get back to the basic question of whether the baby simply has reflux or has reflux disease. In other words, is the baby sick with reflux despite everything we've done? Are there poor weight gain and chronic lung symptoms, for example? If so, the options for treating the baby sick with reflux whose disease doesn't respond to medications get more involved. These cases need the close management expertise of a pediatric gastroenterologist.

For the happy spitter and the gray-zone baby who isn't getting worse, you may simply need to hunker down and recognize that your options are limited. Despite what may be an inconvenience for you, we always have to stay focused on the fact that

"MY BABY INITIALLY DID WELL WITH BETHANECHOL, BUT RECENTLY IT STOPPED WORKING"

Remember that prokinetic medications are prescribed on the basis of a baby's weight, and your baby's weight should change daily. Over time, your baby's medication dosage will need to be adjusted on the basis of her growth. For the baby whose significant reflux responds to prokinetic medications, adjustments in dose may have to be made every 2 to 4 weeks. Growth is one of the most common reasons that medications suddenly "stop working" in infants.

she's not as sick as she could be and her symptoms will decrease with time. Sometimes I address the issue of poorly responsive reflux by helping parents adjust their expectations. For some parents, the idea of frequent spitting up is something that they feel is very abnormal. But despite how they may feel and their desire to have clean carpets, my job is to help them develop realistic expectations. Education is what I do with families who expect something different from what their baby is delivering.

Reflux in the bundle of misery will most often respond in some way to acid-suppression therapy. Parents will sometimes report only a 50% improvement in their baby's screaming with therapy. For many, this change from miserable to fussy is a welcome relief. For other parents, expectations are high and anything less than a perfectly content baby is not enough. Regardless of how little your baby's behavior may turn around, keep in mind that she's suffering with what is typically a self-limited condition. Your baby's reflux will decrease progressively from when she is 4 months of age until she is 12 months of age.

In pediatrics, we find ourselves asking the very important question: "Who are we treating?" And the reality is that while we treat babies, we're also responsible for the parents who care for them. Truth be told, we sometimes order tests to allay the consuming anxiety and fear of a parent. When there's potential benefit and the risks are low, medications can occasionally play as much of a role for parents as they do for a child. If you're the demanding parent of a happy spitter, you need to ask yourself if your interest in changing things is a reflection of your concern for the health of your baby or of your own anxiety.

PUTTING A WRAP ON THINGS—
SURGICAL THERAPY FOR REFLUX

When the best combinations of the best medications prescribed by the best pediatric gastroenterologist don't work and a baby is still sick, the best option is often surgery. Fortunately, this option is rumored, questioned, and discussed far more often than it's actually done. Babies and young children considered candidates for antireflux surgery are typically those with severe reflux complications involving breathing or feeding and growth. Given that this represents major abdominal surgery, physicians do everything in their power to avoid it, especially because we know that reflux in infants decreases over time. Those babies for whom an operation is ultimately recommended represent those with a very low likelihood of ever getting better on their own.

The surgical procedure used to correct severe reflux is called a *fundoplication*. During a fundoplication, part of the top of the stomach (the *fundus*) is wrapped around the lower part of the esophagus and stitched together (or *plicated*). This tighten-

PUT A BIB ON 'EM AND KEEP GOIN'

It's interesting how the expectations of what's acceptable in a baby's behavior vary so widely from family to family. I regularly see happy spitters whose parents insist, "This is *not* normal and something *must* be done." I contrast this with the outlook of my Italian sister-in-law from New Jersey who's never shy about sharing her opinions on matters of child rearing. When I told her that I was writing a book on reflux, she quipped, "What for? You put a bib on 'em and keep goin'. There's nothing you can do about it." While I can't say that I agree with her 100%, there is something to be said for adjusting your expectations and moving on with your life. Reflux can sometimes be controlled to only a certain degree, after which point you have a responsibility to adapt to your baby.

ing of the lower part of the esophagus helps hold stomach contents where they belong.

When this option is suggested, parents will usually show up at the next office visit with a list of questions. This section discusses the seven most common questions that I've fielded from parents regarding fundoplication.

Can This Surgery Be Done Through an Endoscope?

A fundoplication in a child is performed by a pediatric surgeon and can be done in the traditional way through an incision or through a laparoscope. During an open fundoplication, a vertical incision is made in the middle of the abdomen, just below the bottom of the sternum (the breastbone).

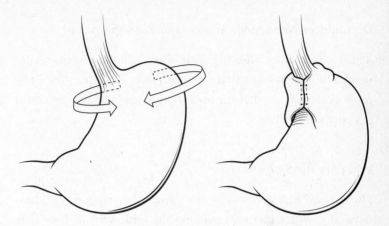

**A fundoplication tightens the connection
between the stomach and the esophagus.**

A laparoscope is a rigid instrument inserted through a tiny incision in a child's abdomen. Two or three laparoscopes are inserted during a typical fundoplication. Air is infused around the organs to allow the surgeon to see. The surgeon controls the rods using video monitoring. A variety of instruments can be passed down through the thin rods for cutting, sewing, and control of bleeding.

An endoscope is a flexible fiber-optic instrument used by a pediatric gastroenterologist to look at the lining of a child's intestine. Endoscopes are passed through the mouth or the anus, and no cutting is involved. There are channels for biopsy forceps and other instruments to allow limited procedures such as controlling bleeding or removing coins and other foreign objects. While antireflux surgery using endoscopy has been done in some cases in adults, this is very experimental in children and isn't recommended by most experts.

Do Children Need Medications After Fundoplication?

There are studies showing that some children occasionally need acid-suppression therapy even after fundoplication, but most experts agree that the operation tends to be very effective at controlling reflux.

What Are the Side Effects?

During the first few weeks after antireflux surgery, children normally will experience some pain with swallowing. This tends to go away as their surgery site heals. Side effects that last beyond the first few weeks after surgery are uncommon but include

- *Gas bloat syndrome:* In this case, children are effectively unable to burp, so they experience painful distention in the upper abdomen, especially after eating. When it doesn't go away on its own, it's sometimes treated with stretching of the fundoplication wrap.
- *Dumping syndrome:* Children with dumping syndrome experience symptoms after eating that include bloating, diarrhea, sweating, and clamminess. These symptoms occur because the stomach is emptying very quickly. The rapid release of carbohydrates into the small intestine leads to wild swings in blood sugar as well as gassy diarrhea. It's believed that this rare postoperative complication arises from pinching of one of the key nerves responsible for the slow, metered emptying of a child's stomach. Dumping syndrome tends to go away with time, but the symptoms can sometimes last for a few months.

We treat dumping syndrome with diet and medications that slow tummy emptying and allow more controlled release of sugar into the bloodstream.

What Happens If the Child Swallows a Poison or Has a Stomach Bug and Needs to Vomit?

A child's need to vomit is one of the most pressing concerns among parents when considering their children for this procedure. Children can occasionally vomit through their fundoplications, but you shouldn't count on it. And in the event of a bad gastroenteritis, which children get from time to time, you can expect some serious retching instead of vomiting. The poisoning question is a legitimate one, but in the event that this occurs, there are ways to irrigate a child's stomach that don't involve vomiting. Of my many patients who have undergone fundoplication, I haven't seen one yet suffer any serious outcome from overdose or poisoning that couldn't be dealt with.

Remember that when we're contemplating this kind of intervention in a child, we're essentially at the end of our rope as far as their reflux disease is concerned. When we're in that position, it's important to keep in mind that we will have to undertake a little risk to achieve the greater benefit of saving their lungs, helping them grow, or whatever it is that indicates the surgery.

Can Fundoplication Be Reversed?

Theoretically, fundoplication can be reversed, but the need to do so is exceptionally rare. When parents ask about this option, it's typically because of concern about complications. Most of the complications of fundoplication are very uncommon, and when they occur, they can be managed.

Does Fundoplication Ever Need to Be Redone?

Though a fundoplication may last forever, it can potentially "break down" or fall apart. At that point the decision to redo the fundoplication will depend on a child's symptoms.

Can Children Burp After Antireflux Surgery?

A child's ability to burp after a fundoplication is limited. This can be a problem in infancy, when burping represents an important mechanism for babies to rid themselves of extra gas that they take in from air swallowing during crying and feeding. In some parts of the United States, pediatric surgeons routinely place a gastrostomy button into the stomach to act as a pop-off valve for gas that has no way out. A gastrostomy button is an appliance placed through the wall of the abdomen into the stomach, usually to help children feed who can't feed well by mouth.

8

A PARENT'S GUIDE TO TESTS
AND STUDIES

Parents vary in their demands and expectations when their baby is irritable and impossible to feed. And the issue of testing or wanting to know with black-and-white certainty about their baby's problem is a very common one. It may seem strange that a chapter on testing would be placed so far toward the end of a book on reflux. After all, isn't testing the first order of business? Shouldn't we first figure out whether a condition is there or not before we jump into treatment? In reality, this is where it belongs simply because testing may be overrated when it comes to babies with reflux.

REFLUX IS A CLINICAL DIAGNOSIS

Let's complicate matters just a little bit by reminding you what we learned in Chapter 1, "The Truth About Crying Babies": All babies have reflux. So when parents ask if their baby has reflux, I can always answer yes. This is the only area in my personal

and professional life where I'm correct 100% of the time. In
fact, I use my smug certainty as a launching point to discuss the
difference between physiologic reflux, which all babies have,
and reflux disease, which is what happens when reflux goes
bad. So the more precise question to ask your physician is "Is
my baby sick from reflux?" or "Are my baby's symptoms possibly attributable to reflux?"

Very well, then. With that technicality resolved, how do we
know if a baby's symptoms are due to reflux? Well, it all goes
back to Chapter 3, "Seven Signs of Reflux in Your Baby." It's
the symptoms we discussed there that tell us with reasonable
certainty whether a child is suffering with reflux. The baby
who comes to my office screaming, congested, hiccupping, spitting up, and taking 40 minutes to consume 3 ounces of formula
or to empty a breast has GER. While this is an oversimplifica-
tion, because other conditions can give a baby some of these
symptoms, most pediatricians and pediatric gastroenterologists
would agree that a baby with these symptoms is most likely
suffering with reflux. GER is a diagnosis that is most frequently made on the basis of a baby's story.

If the Diagnosis of Reflux Is Made on the Basis of a Baby's
Medical History, Why Are There Tests?

You've done Internet searches on it, you've chatted with friends
about it, you've been to your mothers' group where such things
are discussed, and you've heard firsthand about the tests that
can be done. We have the technology, right? Yes, there's no
shortage of technology, but the question is: Who needs it, and
how are we going to use that information? The reality is that
reflux testing isn't something as simple and straightforward as

confirming pregnancy or scanning for gallstones. Unfortunately, there aren't simple, painless, reliable tests for reflux and its complications in babies. Even the most basic studies are relatively invasive, so we have to know that what we're putting a baby through is going to give us information that's going to change her ultimate health outcome.

To Test or Not to Test

If a clinical history is so good, why do we test? Physicians with expertise in treating reflux in children typically consider diagnostic studies when the following questions need to be answered:

- *Are the baby's symptoms due to reflux?* Sometimes babies develop problems that could have a number of causes. Cough or congestion, for example, when severe and unresponsive to simple treatments, can raise suspicions about reflux. But when a baby or young child lacks other symptoms to suggest reflux disease, sometimes we need to confirm it or rule it out. Testing may play a role in the screaming baby who doesn't have typical symptoms of reflux and whose condition hasn't responded to therapy.
- *How bad is the baby's reflux?* Occasionally, we want to know how much reflux a baby has or, if very sick, if they're responding to the therapy that we've prescribed. Testing sometimes lets us know what kind of job we're doing as doctors and parents.
- *Is the baby's reflux causing damage?* If reflux has been going on for a while, we sometimes like to know if a child has sustained any injury to the esophagus. In this case, testing isn't to look for reflux itself necessarily but rather

for its secondary effects. Remember that all babies have reflux, but not all babies have reflux disease. Testing can help sort that out when necessary.

Studies are done when we're unsure that it's reflux, to see how bad it is, or to look for complications. Keep in mind that all that spits is not reflux, so your physician may put your baby through testing that has nothing to do with reflux. If the diagnosis of reflux is in question, you physician may test for other problems such as urinary tract infections, blood chemical imbalances, or anatomic problems in the intestinal tract.

Just as with Allergy, Sometimes Treating Is the Best Test

Sometimes if a physician suspects reflux, she'll go ahead and treat it. If your physician does this, don't be alarmed. It's practical and entirely within the confines of good medical practice. You may recall that this is sometimes the approach with milk allergy in infancy.

TESTING 1, 2, 3 . . .

What kinds of tests can you expect, and what will these tests potentially tell us? We'll talk about three of the more commonly considered tests in the baby with reflux: the upper GI series, endoscopy, and the esophageal pH probe.

Upper Gastrointestinal Series

Looking only at the number of times that spitting, screaming babies are sent to have an upper GI series, one might think that the upper GI series is the granddaddy of reflux tests, the gold standard and end-all for desperate parents and similarly desperate pediatricians. But unfortunately, this is perhaps the most overrated and overused study among babies with reflux.

What Is an Upper Gastrointestinal Series?

An upper GI series is a test used to evaluate the anatomy of the upper intestinal tract. It enables the radiologist to examine the outline of the esophagus, stomach, and upper intestine and to look for congenital malformations, twists, kinks, or other problems that could predispose to vomiting or poor feeding. In other words, the upper GI series is an anatomy test. It tells us if everything is in the right place.

During this test, a child is given a few ounces of a material called barium, which is swallowed from a cup or bottle. The child is then placed under an X-ray machine called a fluoroscope. When images are taken, the barium shows up as stark white, so it allows physicians to see an outline of a child's upper intestinal tract. More specifically, the upper GI series allows visualization of the esophagus, stomach, and small intestine just beyond the stomach. The entire small intestinal tract is not studied with an upper GI series. A typical study in a cooperative child takes no more than a few minutes.

If your child is an independent sort, you may be concerned that he's not going to be willing to drink anything but his own milk from his cup on his terms. This is a common concern and an occasional obstacle to a good upper GI study. But if your physician has referred you to a center that routinely performs this study on children, you'll have the help of radiology technicians with expertise in getting children to do what needs to be done. Barium isn't the best-tasting stuff in the world, so it can be flavored. When the study absolutely has to be done and a child absolutely will not take the barium, syringe feeding is attempted. And in those children who refuse syringe feeding, a tube can be placed through the nose and into the stomach so that the barium can be given that way.

The Upper Gastrointestinal Series Is Not a Reflux Test

The keen observer will note that I've said nothing about reflux in discussing the upper GI series. That's because it isn't a reflux test. Unfortunately, this is one of the most common misconceptions among primary care physicians, and it creates confusion for families. I've heard it a thousand times: A physician sees a baby with symptoms of reflux and comments, "Hmm, spitting and fussiness. Looks like reflux. Let's do an upper GI to see." Though you may be thrilled that your physician is taking some kind of action, you may want to hold your enthusiasm. There are two problems with using the upper GI series as a reflux test:

- All babies have reflux.
- Your baby may not reflux during the few minutes of the test.

If all babies have reflux, seeing it on an upper GI series gives us no new information. And if there isn't a wave of reflux seen during this brief study, it doesn't rule out the fact that caustic acid may be bathing your baby's esophagus during the other 23 hours and 58 minutes of the day.

Deciding Who Needs an Upper Gastrointestinal Series

Despite telling you all the things that an upper GI series won't do, I must say that this test is very good at what it's intended for—namely, looking for anatomic issues that could be responsible for your baby's problems. For some babies with reflux symptoms, the upper GI series is an important test. So which babies would those be? Babies with . . .

- *Vomiting that is forceful:* Babies with even mild reflux can have impressive vomiting from time to time, but the baby with consistently forceful vomiting should have obstructive problems ruled out with an upper GI series. Most folks would consider forceful vomiting to be vomit that shoots from a baby's mouth.
- *Reflux with complications:* Babies with reflux that keeps them from gaining the weight that they should are candidates for an upper GI series. In general, babies who are truly sick from their reflux should have anatomic problems eliminated as a possibility.
- *Feeding problems:* While difficulty breastfeeding or bottle-feeding is one of the hallmarks of reflux esophagitis, it can be due to congenital blockages in the esophagus and stomach. When it doesn't seem like garden-variety reflux, your physician may consider an upper GI series.
- *Reflux that won't go away:* Some doctors will give a baby time to allow symptoms to decrease, because we know that most do when given time. But as a baby gets into the later part of her first year and shows no signs of improvement, it may be reasonable to look to see if everything is in place anatomically.

The upper GI series can be helpful in allowing us to view the anatomy of the intestines, but it's unable to tell us what's going on in the lining of the intestine. This is where endoscopy comes in.

Endoscopy—Seeing Your Baby from the Inside Out

When parents learn a little bit about reflux and recognize what it can potentially do to their children, they often start asking questions such as "How do I know that my baby's reflux hasn't caused damage?" And this is where endoscopy can play a role in caring for the child with reflux.

What Is Endoscopy?

Endoscopy is the tool used by pediatric gastroenterologists to look at the inside of a child's intestinal tract. It is performed with a thin, flexible fiber-optic camera that can be passed into the mouth or anus to look at the lining of the intestinal tract for problems. Beyond just looking for problems, endoscopy can be used for therapeutic purposes such as stopping bleeding and removing polyps when necessary. When we're specifically concerned about reflux and its complications, *upper endoscopy* is performed. This is commonly referred to as an EGD (esophagogastroduodenoscopy).

During an EGD, a gastroenterologist passes an endoscope through the mouth, down the esophagus, into the stomach, and beyond to the small intestine. The lining of the esophagus is carefully inspected, with attention focused on any injury that may have occurred from reflux. Evaluation of the stomach and upper small intestine sometimes gives clues as to why a child has such slow tummy emptying or so much vomiting. And sometimes an EGD doesn't show much at all.

As you might imagine, this isn't a test that can be done on kids while they're awake. Endoscopy in children is typically done with either general anesthesia or heavy sedation. You'll notice that your physician will recommend that your child not

IS THAT A SCOPE, SCAN, SERIES, OR SWALLOW?

Some of the studies physicians order to evaluate refluxing children can get confusing. Here's the nitty-gritty on what's what for some of the different barium X-ray studies you may encounter:

- *Upper GI series:* Looks at the esophagus, stomach, and upper small intestine. This is the gold standard for looking for anatomic problems in vomiting children.

- *Upper GI series with small bowel series:* This is an upper GI series that goes beyond the upper small intestine to look at the outline of the entire small intestine. It takes much longer than a simple upper GI series and may be less helpful in evaluating vomiting children.

- *Esophogram:* This is essentially a barium study that looks only at the esophagus. It's used when we're interested in seeing only the esophagus to rule out narrowing of the esophagus or the presence of foreign objects, such as plastic toys that can be ingested by inquisitive children.

- *Swallow study:* The swallow function study evaluates how kids handle different kinds of foods. During this study, children are given thin liquid, thickened liquid, and solid food to see how it is swallowed. The mechanics of bolus formation and swallowing are followed on X-ray. It's helpful when we want to make sure certain foods aren't going into the lungs. Neurologic and anatomic swallowing problems can be identified with a swallow study.

- *Barium swallow:* Technically, this is the same as an esophogram, although sometimes you'll hear the term used loosely for upper GI studies and sometimes even swallow studies.

> ### WHAT HAPPENS IF SHE THROWS UP THE STUFF THAT WE'RE GIVING HER TO SEE WHY SHE'S THROWING UP?
>
> As you might expect, your baby may throw up during her upper GI series. But babies sometimes retain enough barium to allow the radiologist to see what needs to be seen. If that isn't the case, more barium can always be given to your baby to complete the study.

eat or drink for 4 to 6 hours before her endoscopy. Part of the reason for this preparation is the obvious difficulty that physicians would have navigating around a tummy full of food residue. The other important reason kids can't eat before endoscopy is the risk of the sedation itself. When children are sleepy, their ability to naturally protect their windpipe from vomit is impaired, so keeping the tummy empty helps prevent frightening breathing complications.

During an EGD, small pinches of tissue called biopsies are usually taken. When parents hear *biopsy*, they often think cancer, but this means nothing more than a tissue sample. The biopsies taken give physicians valuable information about the extent of injury a child may have sustained in the esophagus. Biopsies in the stomach and upper intestine help us diagnose conditions such as allergy that can give a child refluxlike symptoms. Your physician will most likely take some pictures for the record. These are helpful for comparison when endoscopic follow-up is necessary.

Deciding Who Needs an EGD

You may be thinking at this point: *Hmm, this sounds like just the test for my bundle of misery ... look for evidence of acid re-*

WHAT TO EXPECT: UPPER GASTROINTESTINAL SERIES

- *Length of time:* 15 to 30 minutes
- *Before:* Nothing to eat for 4 to 6 hours
- *Intravenous (IV) tube:* No
- *Sedation:* No
- *Recovery:* Home immediately after completing the study
- *After:* Offer plenty of fluid to flush out barium, which can harden and cause bad constipation

---

flux damage and make a diagnosis. Sign me up. Not so fast. While endoscopy is an important tool in the management of some cases of reflux, it is necessary in only a small number of cases, especially in babies. So who needs a look? Upper endoscopy will help . . .

- *Tell reflux from allergy:* As we've learned, reflux and milk protein allergy represent two of the most common reasons for babies to scream inconsolably. When babies with intractable screaming don't get better with reflux therapy, endoscopy may play a role in figuring out what's going on. Looking at the lining of a baby's intestinal tract and taking biopsies usually allow a pediatric gastroenterologist to tell these two problems apart. And sometimes finding nothing gives us as much information as anything.
- *Define the extent of reflux injury in a child with reflux complications:* I did just say that we sometimes look to tell reflux from allergy, but remember that it's entirely appropriate for a physician to treat for these conditions without

first looking at your baby's innards. It's just that when babies are sick with poor growth, lung complications, or severe feeding difficulty, we sometimes like to get a "tissue diagnosis" to waste as little time as possible starting the right therapy. And parents are usually on board with this strategy because they're the ones living with the baby.

In the child whom we know has had reflux for some months, endoscopy helps us determine whether there has been any injury and its extent. A good example of this is the child with reflux as an infant who moves into toddlerhood without growing out of her reflux. Depending on the extent of her symptoms, a pediatric gastroenterologist may want to survey the esophagus to exclude the possibility of chronic esophagitis. In the child with chronic asthma and reflux, an endoscope may help define the extent of reflux and help change the direction of therapy for their lung disease.

- *Evaluate unexplained feeding difficulty:* Babies with difficulty feeding or toddlers and young children with painful swallowing are often evaluated endoscopically to look for reflux. Other conditions such as infections of the esophagus can be identified through an endoscope.
- *Explain unexplained vomiting:* When a child's vomiting isn't easily explained and anatomic anomalies have been excluded by upper GI series, a look at the upper intestinal tract is often the next study done.

Ultimately, your pediatric gastroenterologist will determine whether your child is a candidate for endoscopy. As a general rule, most babies with reflux can be monitored and treated without ever considering endoscopy.

WHAT TO EXPECT: EGD

- *Length of time:* 10 to 30 minutes for the procedure itself, but expect to spend half a day from preparation to recovery
- *Before:* Nothing to eat for 4 to 6 hours
- *IV tube:* Yes
- *Sedation:* Yes
- *Recovery:* Observation for about an hour, grogginess for several hours; when the child is awake and can hold his head up, he can drink; when he can drink, he can eat
- *After:* Expect some flatulence from air used during the procedure; be sure to ask your physician for copies of pictures taken in your child's tummy

---

pH Probe

Surely there must be a test for reflux better than what we've already talked about. Let's talk about a test that's been designed solely and exclusively for telling whether someone has reflux and how much of it they've got. But though it may seem like the gold standard in reflux testing, it isn't always necessary in the baby with reflux.

What Is a pH Probe?

Testing with a pH probe allows physicians to see just how much reflux a child is having and when they're having it. During this study, a small, spaghetti-like tube is placed through the nose and down into the esophagus, where it remains for 24 hours. At the esophagus end of the tube is a very tiny sensor that can detect changes in a child's acid level—or pH changes—in the esophagus. The outside end of the tube is attached to a little recording device about the size of an iPod audio player. As reflux occurs during the course of the test, information is sent to a recording device, where it is stored and later downloaded for review by a pediatric gastroenterologist. During the test, the parent keeps a detailed diary of significant events that go on, such as choking, coughing, screaming, and feeding. This diary can then be compared with the reflux activity that's recorded.

Done over a 24-hour period, a pH probe study allows a pediatric gastroenterologist to see

- When reflux occurs
- How long reflux episodes last
- The total amount of time that the child refluxes in a day
- If reflux corresponds to other problems noted by the parent

This information is then interpreted within the context of a child's symptoms and used to help guide therapy.

Deciding Who Needs a pH Probe

A pH probe sounds like a great way to tell if your child has reflux. It is, but it may not be necessary. Remember that reflux is a diagnosis typically based on a child's medical history. A trained physician can listen to a child's symptoms and, with reasonable accuracy, determine whether reflux is a problem. But sometimes this is easier said than done. Take, for example, the following scenarios:

- A 2-month-old has seizurelike head movements and normal findings on a brainwave scan. There are no obvious symptoms of reflux to explain his movements as a manifestation of esophagitis.

- An 18-month-old with reflux as an infant, now apparently resolved, awakens every night screaming and arching. There are no other symptoms of reflux, and it doesn't seem like behavioral awakening.
- A 9-month-old has a chronic cough and wheezing that doesn't respond well to typical medications. There are no other symptoms to suggest reflux.

In each of these cases (and you may need to take my word for it), there isn't clear evidence of reflux when the child is examined at an office visit. But in each of these cases, reflux could easily be the culprit. The pediatric gastroenterologist who finds himself in this predicament finds solace in the pH probe, which can help him to prove that significant reflux is present. The pH probe also tells us that reflux is occurring at the time when the child is experiencing her worst symptoms.

Esophageal pH Studies—Not Always the Golden Egg
Even in the situations mentioned previously, the pH probe may not be all that it's cracked up to be. I hate to sound like a broken record, but remember that reflux is a normal physiologic event seen in all babies and children. And we see this on pH probe studies. Kids have lots of mini blips of acid that come up and are short-lived. They have a very characteristic appearance on pH probe studies. They are very normal.

But some of these very normal physiologic blips of acid can create big problems that aren't always easy to pick up. These tiny, normal-appearing events can sometimes lead to minute amounts of acid entering the upper airway, leading to wheezing and coughing. Sometimes such small reflux events can even make a baby hold her breath and change color for a short time. However, proving that these apparently normal physiologic reflux events are the cause of a baby's problem can be difficult, so the decision of when to perform an esophageal pH study and understanding how to interpret it takes a great deal of experience as well as an intimate understanding of the child's symptoms.

As sketchy as it may seem in some cases, the pH probe remains our best hope for picking up reflux in the child when we're not sure it's there.

Gastric Emptying Scan/Nuclear Scintiscan

Upper GI series, scopes, and probes make up the core of testing that young children may undergo for reflux. But as you can imagine, there are other ways to evaluate the young child when we're suspicious about reflux and its complications. We'll talk about one called the gastric emptying scan, but don't expect it to be on your pediatrician's short list of things to do for your child. This less frequently used diagnostic study can shine in certain circumstances, but its use is very specific.

What Is a Gastric Emptying Scan?
We've said that one of the problems behind reflux is poor tummy emptying. How can we tell this is a problem in a child? A study called a gastric emptying scan measures how long it takes for the stomach to empty. During this test, a small amount of low-level, short-acting radioactive tracer is put into milk or food and fed to the child. The child is then put in front

"HOW DO YOU GET A TWELVE-MONTH-OLD TO KEEP A TUBE IN HIS NOSE?"

When I discuss the possibility of a pH probe with parents, the first question out of their mouths concerns keeping the tube in. That's understandable because infants and toddlers have a hard time following directions. Surprisingly, it's less of a problem than you'd think. The urge to pull and pick tends to come from the irritation of the tape used to secure a pH probe. When the tube is secured soundly in place by an experienced pediatric nurse, kids usually leave them alone. More often the probe is hooked or caught on the fingers by mistake. You may be given arm restraints that keep a child's elbows straight and his hands unable to cause trouble. Watch your child and use these if you must. But often the concern in this case is greater than the problem itself.

of a scanner that can show the tracer activity in the stomach. Periodically over the course of an hour or two, the child is re-scanned to see how much of the original material is remaining in the stomach. It's actually an interesting test to watch because you can see what amounts to a blob of food in the stomach at the start of the study that (hopefully) moves with each subsequent scan. With the assistance of sophisticated software and experienced nuclear medicine physicians, a child's gastric emptying time can be calculated and compared to what's normal.

We can often identify delayed tummy emptying in a child from the medical history alone, but the gastric emptying scan is helpful when it absolutely has to be proven. Sometimes this

WHAT TO EXPECT: pH PROBE

- *Length of time:* 24 hours
- *Before:* Nothing to eat for 4 to 6 hours; no acid suppressants for at least 48 hours before the study
- *IV tube:* None
- *Sedation:* Typically not used
- *Recovery:* Fussiness for a few minutes after the probe goes in; after that, it's business as usual—children eat and drink as they normally would
- *After:* Nothing special

is necessary when contemplating a fundoplication because a severe gastric emptying delay in a child could be a predictor of problems after surgery. And like so many of our tummy studies, the gastric emptying scan can sometimes help us make sense of symptoms that don't seem to make sense.

Using Nuclear Medicine to Diagnose Reflux
The same technology used to follow gastric emptying can be used to look for reflux. When tracer material is given along with a baby's meal, it's possible to follow it to see where it winds up. Sometimes this is referred to as a *nuclear scintiscan*. Specifically, this test gives physicians the opportunity to see if the stuff initially in the stomach has made its way up the esophagus to other places like the lungs. Difficult-to-identify aspiration (remember from Chapter 3, "Seven Signs of Reflux in Your Baby," that this is when stuff comes up and goes into the lungs) can be picked up with this test. It also comes in

HOW LONG SHOULD IT TAKE THE TUMMY TO EMPTY?

How long does milk or baby food hang out in a baby's stomach after it's eaten? The body handles liquids and solids differently. In general, we can expect water to empty from the stomach in 30 minutes, milk in 60 minutes, and solids in about 90 minutes. These numbers vary widely depending on what's eaten, what it's eaten with, and how much is eaten. And remember that delayed tummy emptying is common in babies with reflux.

handy when looking for reflux in children who have had antireflux surgery but still have symptoms suggestive of reflux.

BE AN EDUCATED HEALTH CARE CONSUMER

Getting testing is sometimes easier said than done when it comes to kids. Depending on where you live, accessibility to the proper resources may be difficult. And the tools your physician has at her disposal may figure into how your child is treated. In other words, physicians practicing in small, rural communities may not be able to order an esophageal pH study or gastric emptying scan even if they want to. As you know by now, however, this shouldn't create too much of a problem for most babies with reflux because testing doesn't play a big role in diagnosis and therapy.

But if your baby is sick and she does need more attention than the average bear, there are some things you should know. Specifically, not all facilities are created equal when it comes to little tykes. A study done in one hospital may not be performed at the same level of expertise as in another hospital. A test can have different results when done by different physicians. That shouldn't be the case, but unfortunately it can be. Education is your best assurance that your child gets the best care possible.

If your child requires any special testing for reflux, be sure to insist on a facility that routinely treats children. This point is more important in very young and sick babies. Children are different from adults in that they can require a great deal of care and attention just to successfully complete some of these tests we've talked about. Any facility can muddle through a diagnostic test with a screaming baby and generate a report, but what physicians need to see is a thorough, well-done study that answers the questions we have about their condition.

Your physician will give you guidance, but be sure to ask the right questions. Here's what you should know up front:

Know the Facility Doing Your Child's Test

Many hospitals will agree to take a crack at a child, but your child needs to be tested at a facility that routinely deals with sick children. Not only will the results of your child's evaluation be more reliable in such a place but also your experience and that of your child will be very different than in a less specialized facility. Look to your region's children's hospital for the best care tailored to kids. Small community hospitals vary considerably when it comes to providing reliable care to small children, so be sure to check them out. Avoid "supermarket" or chain radiology centers that are often found in communities. They may seem convenient, but you could be wasting your time.

Know About the Physicians Doing Your Child's Test

Look to your child's physician for advice, but remember that children are always better off being treated by physicians used to dealing with children.

- If your child needs an upper GI series, ask if your child's test is going to be performed and interpreted by a pediatric radiologist. Small babies have to be held in just the right spot to look for positioning problems in the intestinal tract. Facilities without technicians skilled in the proper positioning techniques often fail to get complete upper GI studies. If pediatric radiologists are nowhere to be found, inquire if the radiologists conducting your child's test are accustomed to working with babies.
- If your child is having a pH probe, check to be sure that it will be interpreted by a board-certified pediatric gastroenterologist. The law allows neonatologists and other specialists to collect a fee for trying to read pH probes, but they're not trained to do so.
- If your child is having endoscopy with anesthesia, a pediatric anesthesiologist is preferred in the event of complications. Insist at a very minimum that a physician be present at all times with your child while she is under anesthesia. Many facilities staff their operating rooms with less well paid nurse anesthetists, who may have very limited experience in pediatrics, to cut costs. Don't let your child be on the receiving end of a cost-containment measure. If you insist on the presence of a physician, the facility will likely comply rather than lose your business.

If the facility refuses, consider looking somewhere else for your care.

Try to do your investigating before committing your child to any type of procedure. There's nothing worse than keeping your child without food until the middle of the morning only to decide that the facility isn't the best for your child.

Put Convenience Aside

Understand that the services that your child needs may not be available in your immediate area. If this is the case, it's in the best interest of your child to travel an extra hour or two to a facility that can provide you with reliable testing rather than undergo a bad experience and get fuzzy results.

For many parents the idea of testing is a preoccupation based on misconceptions. Despite technological advances, reflux may be tricky to put our finger on, and testing may not even be necessary. Though your physician is the expert, you're ultimately your child's best advocate. The questions you ask and the decisions you make will influence the care your child gets.

9

WHAT TO EXPECT FROM YOUR PHYSICIAN

YOUR PHYSICIAN: KEY TO YOUR BABY'S HAPPINESS OR PART OF THE PROBLEM?

In the 1960s it was said that if you weren't part of the solution, you were part of the problem. And in some respects, we could say the same thing about your physician's view of infant irritability today. At the dawn of the twenty-first century, there's evidence to suggest that many of the miserable babies that we once believed had a mysterious condition referred to as colic actually are living with one or more treatable conditions.

But you're a parent and she's the doctor, right? True, but today, health care is a consumer-driven commodity. If we don't like the care that we're given, we can simply move on and choose the care that we wish. This can be a good thing because we, as patients and parents, are empowered with information that allows us to assess whether the care that we're receiving is

BABY GEORGE: ANTIDEPRESSANTS VERSUS ANTACIDS FOR REFLUX

"I'll never forget my first child, George, and how he screamed for the first 5 months of his life. Our family physician at the time suggested that I take an antidepressant—something about adjusting to George. Only recently when our second baby showed all of the exact symptoms that George had had and stopped screaming with reflux treatment did I realize that it wasn't me. I didn't have anything wrong with me. My baby really was sick."

reasonable. We're just a few clicks away from knowing everything about our physician's history. We can even find rankings of our physician's competence.

But we have to understand that with this power comes responsibility. We have to understand that we have a responsibility to our babies to recognize our limits. Rather than believe that we can go it alone, we have to fashion an understanding of our role and that of our physician in our baby's care. As part of this new world, you can ask questions and should expect answers. So what should you expect from your physician?

Picking Your Provider

All kinds of different providers care for babies. Most common among these are pediatricians, family practitioners, and allied clinicians such as nurse practitioners and physician assistants. In fact, you may be surprised to learn that in most states, anyone who holds a valid medical license can prescribe medications for tiny babies.

Your access to specialists or even certain kinds of primary care physicians may be dictated by where you live, so you might not even have much choice. In rural parts of the United States, for example, care for folks of all ages is provided by family practitioners, and pediatricians may be considered a scarcity. In large metropolitan areas, by contrast, abundant numbers of pediatricians make them the standard health care providers for babies and tots. The way that screaming babies are cared for in these areas may be influenced by the ready availability of pediatric gastroenterologists. Sometimes when faced with a bundle of misery and a couple of miserable parents, pediatricians will look to a gastroenterologist for help sooner rather than later. This isn't always necessary, but the stress brought on by a screaming bundle will often force the use of all available resources.

While to some families an M.D. is an M.D., not all are trained the same way. Pediatricians spend 3 years after medical school in residency, training in caring only for children. Normal nursery care, neonatal intensive medicine, and subspecialty rotations prepare pediatricians to care for the tiniest patients. Family practitioners also spend 3 years after medical school in residency. But their residency training covers all ages during that period, and the amount of time learning baby medicine is quite limited when compared with a residency dedicated solely to kids.

The bottom line is that when your baby is miserable and not headed in the right direction, I first recommend seeking out the input of the most trained individual in your area, and in most cases that person is a board-certified pediatrician.

Is Your Pediatrician Up for Treating Reflux?

Now more than ever, pediatricians should be aware of the signs of pediatric GER and its treatment. In 2001 the NASPGHAN published GERD practice guidelines to give pediatricians some idea of how to handle refluxing babies. This was followed by an aggressive public education campaign to raise awareness among parents and pediatricians. But despite efforts to bring America's pediatricians up to speed with reflux care, there is still work to be done. According to a 2005 study of the knowledge, attitudes, and practice styles of North American pediatricians regarding reflux, more than 75% of pediatricians weren't aware that there are published guidelines for reflux care in children.

So is your physician up to the task of treating your baby's reflux? The short answer is: She should be. But as we can see from the statistics, the longer answer is that some aren't in the habit of recognizing reflux. And when you're not used to diagnosing it, you're probably not on your game when it comes to treating it. As time passes and the training of physicians improves, young pediatricians coming out of residency are less inclined to blame parents as "overwhelmed" and more apt to recognize that there are identifiable and treatable causes of profound irritability in babies.

So How Can You Tell If You're Dealing with Someone Who's on Board?

Getting care for your baby with reflux is a lot like getting your car repaired. You never really know if mechanics have any idea of what they're doing, and the funny noises that your car has

SIGNS OF A GOOD PEDIATRICIAN

Too little time and not enough money has some physicians cutting kids short. This is what to look for in a good pediatrician:

- Takes a thorough medical history and does a thorough exam
- Considers all possibilities
- Doesn't jump to quick conclusions
- Has excellent judgment
- Has a plan of attack
- Is up-to-date on all of the latest treatments

been making for days always seem to disappear when you drive into the shop. And so it goes for babies.

Despite how many books you've read, it may be hard to know if the care that your baby is getting is the best care she can get. Your ability as a health care consumer to judge the quality of something as specific and specialized as infant medicine is limited. But this is no excuse for not trying. There are some things you can do to maximize the odds that what needs to get done will be done.

Ask Questions and Expect Answers

Parents who come prepared and informed command more of a physician's attention than those who don't. The best thing you can do to ensure that your baby gets the attention she deserves is to be informed.

Look for flexibility and willingness to consider all options. In the twentieth-century paternalistic model of the physician–patient relationship, parents did as they were told and that was that. But an intelligent, experienced pediatrician in the twenty-first century understands that with babies, things may not always be what they seem. Flexibility and an open-minded approach will create opportunities to try options that may help your baby.

Watch for the C Word

If your baby's physician comes up with the "diagnosis" of colic, you should be suspicious. Remember that colic is just a catch-all, a place for us to hide when there's nowhere else to go and no more answers to be had. If your physician uses the C word, ask some questions:

- How can we be sure my baby doesn't have reflux?
- How can we be sure that my baby isn't suffering with milk protein allergy?
- If we don't have other options, can we consider treating for either of these conditions because their appearance in babies can look like "colic"?

The answer you get should reflect that these are reasonable considerations. If your physician believes that empiric treatment is either not indicated or even contraindicated for your baby, ask questions to understand why. Every baby is different and each has to be treated individually.

Be on the Lookout for Excessive Testing

Remember that reflux is a clinical diagnosis and testing usually does little to change the outcome for the typical baby with reflux (see Chapter 6, "The Care and Handling of Your Crying,

Spitting, Difficult-to-Soothe Baby"). Always ask how testing is going to change what's ultimately done for your baby. If you're unsure about the necessity of a test, get another opinion.

If Your Physician Is Outdated, Outwitted, or Intimidated, Find Another Physician

You need a physician who's going to confidently approach your child's irritability in a systematic way that involves considering all options. Expect a plan, an endpoint, and a contingency plan if your child's condition doesn't improve. Be suspicious if there isn't some semblance of a plan.

If your baby's symptoms match what you read about in Chapter 3 ("Seven Signs of Reflux in Your Baby") and your concerns are dismissed by your physicians, it may be time to look elsewhere. Disregard for you and your baby is never acceptable, and you deserve better.

Sometimes a physician's approach with irritable babies is to keep the parents busy with tactics and maneuvers that do more to buy time than give relief. Wrapping and shushing have their role in settling every baby, but maneuvers such as these probably do a better job of keeping parents busy than making truly miserable babies feel better. And if your physician's too busy to explain what's being done and why, it may be time to find another physician. If you choose to get a second opinion, you might look for a pediatrician who has only recently completed his or her training. Younger doctors are often better trained at recognizing reflux disease for what it is.

Talk to Other Parents

Talk to other parents to find out who among local pediatricians listens, who spends the time, and who's flexible as far as considering new ways of thinking. Networking among other parents is one of the best ways to ensure that you hook up with a good physician.

MAKING THE MOST OF YOUR TIME WITH THE PHYSICIAN

Your Relationship with Your Pediatrician Is Just That . . . a Relationship

I learned a lot from one particular screaming baby early on in my practice. The mother called me in exhausted desperation one evening, saying that the only thing keeping her daughter happy was the sound of the vacuum cleaner. I couldn't resist and quipped something about how wonderfully clean the house must be. She immediately broke into tears and hung up on me. I felt terrible about my brash insensitivity and called back right away to apologize. With my admission of guilt, she went on to admit that she too was on edge. We laughed a bit, and everything was fine after that. At the time, my wife and I were childless and the true impact of an intractably irritable baby was something foreign to me. I learned that evening, and subsequently with my own wife, to never mess with a tired mother.

Sometimes, as physicians, we fail to understand where our patients are at when they're tired and desperate. And sometimes as parents we fail to remember that pediatricians are human and that the stress and pressure of dealing with desperate families all day long can be overwhelming. Physicians, like parents, can be tired and stressed. It must be clear to patients and physicians alike that the encounters between a physician and patient very much constitute a relationship. It's no differ-

BE SUSPICIOUS WHEN YOUR PHYSICIAN SUGGESTS DISCONTINUING BREASTFEEDING

Many times the first impulse when dealing with a screaming baby is to pull the breast milk. Be suspicious of anyone who suggests this up front. For reflux this may not be such a good idea, and as we learned in Chapter 6 ("The Care and Handling of Your Crying, Spitting, Difficult-to-Soothe Baby"), allergic breastfed babies can usually continue to breastfeed with modifications to Mom's diet. The only time that cessation of breastfeeding is potentially warranted is in cases of severe allergy or in a dangerously ill baby where intake is in question. Even in this latter case, expressed breast milk can be supplemented to higher caloric density and given via a feeding tube.

ent from any other relationship, be it friendship, marriage, or business.

Aaron Lazare, M.D., my psychiatry professor at the University of Massachusetts Medical School in the 1980s, taught that negotiation is key to every physician–patient encounter. That message is one that the consumer-patient of the new millennium needs to hear too. As patients and parents, we all have a commitment to our relationships with our physicians. This isn't the typical advice that you might find in a parenting book, but I suggest that it's in the best interest of your baby that you always keep your physician's position in the back of your mind. This realistic recognition of your physician's own frailties is important in ultimately getting your baby the care that she needs.

PHYSICIANS AND OTHER HEALTH CARE PROVIDERS

Before you dole out respect to your physician, you may want to make sure you're talking to one. The latest trend among busy medical practices is to hire pediatric nurse practitioners and physician assistants to handle the heavy lifting and heavy volumes. Some offices have even adopted the shady practice of referring to their nurse clinicians as doctors. (Often the masquerade will involve sticking *Dr.* in front of the clinicians' first name.) While allied clinicians are fantastic at handling the basics, remember that your little bundle of misery is only a step away from seeing a pediatric subspecialist. Ask questions, don't be embarrassed, and insist on seeing a physician.

Building a Healthy Relationship with Your Pediatrician: Eight Do's and Don'ts for Getting Taken Seriously with a Miserable Baby

What can you do to make your relationship with your physician healthier? Here are a few tips:

- *She's the doctor, so give her a little respect too.* The Internet has us all thinking that we're experts, but always remember that your baby's physician is still someone with years of training. She deserves to be treated with some respect.
- *Remember that your physician has other patients.* You do need to state your case, but be sure to do it concisely. Understand that despite your feeling that the physician should devote her whole afternoon to you, this will never

A LITTLE RESPECT

You may be convinced that you're a neurotic parent, but no one is in a position to judge a sleep-deprived, stressed-out parent with a screaming baby. It's your responsibility to make your case for your baby, but it's your physician's responsibility to take your situation seriously. Don't let your physician's office staff members put you off, and don't be afraid to look elsewhere if you're not getting the attention you deserve.

happen. Make good use of your time by preparing your case and knowing your questions. Write them down to be sure you cover everything. And consider bringing your spouse or a relative for support or help should the baby begin screaming. There's nothing more frustrating for a physician than trying to discuss a plan of care while a baby begins stating her own case. And one last thing: Be on time even though there's no guarantee your physician will be!

- *Make your agenda clear.* One of the sources of frustration in the physician–parent relationship is a difference in expectations. Physicians are trying to make sure babies don't have anything life-threatening going on. Parents are often just looking for a little relief. Both of these are reasonable goals, but often one party isn't aware of the other's intention. If your gray-zone baby looks rosy in the office, it's up to you to make it clear that your baby is struggling to feed and you're struggling to maintain your sanity. Make your feelings known. Let the physician know what you're going through and state your case.

- *Never exaggerate your child's condition.* One way to get off on the wrong foot is to exaggerate your baby's condition. If you have to exaggerate to get attention, you're either stating your case incorrectly or you're not being listened to. Confidently convey what's going on and look for an interested, empathetic response.

- *As hard as it may be, be patient.* Remember that treating reflux is like steering a boat. You have to give your physician the time to let a treatment plan work.

- *Be realistic.* Reflux is a normal, physiologic condition and sometimes in babies it can be corrected only to a certain point. While how far you go with the treatment of your baby should be a point of negotiation between you and your physician, be realistic about your expectations. Just keep in mind that pediatricians serve two customers: parents and babies. The decisions that your physician makes may better benefit your baby than you.

- *Recognize your own level of stress.* Sometimes your sense of urgency is an important tool in getting the attention you need, but it can easily get out of control. Despite your mind-numbing fatigue, try to hold it together in the interest of your baby. Remember that the relationship you share with your pediatrician may ultimately affect your baby's care.

- *Make sure you're barking up the right tree.* If your physician has referred you to a specialist, then that's whom you should be talking to. Once a pediatrician has made a referral for help with the miserable baby, she's reached her limit on what she can offer. Be sure you're talking to the right person. If you're involved with a pediatric gastroenterologist, that's probably who you should be calling.

DON'T MESS WITH THE GATEKEEPER

Whatever you do, don't diss the office staff. And never refuse to discuss your child's case with the nurse. You may feel your situation is urgent, but your pediatrician's practice has lots of parents with urgent situations who would love to speak immediately with the physician. Nurse triage is a key step to determining how important a child's problem is. Don't interfere with it.

What Kind of Information Do You Need to Be Sure to Get from the Physician?

Part of your job as a parent is to be sure that you take away what you need to know when consulting your pediatrician or pediatric gastroenterologist:

- *The diagnosis:* What's the working diagnosis, and what's being treated? It's important to know the direction your physician is taking. Don't be surprised if your physician doesn't have a firm diagnosis. Often the best physicians don't jump to quick conclusions but rather will create a short list of possibilities, referred to as a *differential diagnosis.*
- *The plan:* Ask what's next if the prescribed plan doesn't work. Your physician should be able to offer a contingency plan that is based on the differential diagnosis.
- *The dosage:* Confirm the dosages of prescribed medications.
- *The length of follow-up:* Confirm close follow-up with your doctor. Your bundle of misery shouldn't have to wait 6 weeks for a follow-up visit. Depending on her level of irritability, weight gain, and the planned intervention, you

should expect follow-up in 2 to 3 weeks at the most. If weight gain is a problem in your refluxing baby, most physicians will want to see you back within a week.

- *The prep:* If tests are planned, be sure that you have the proper instructions for preparing your baby: How long does he need to fast, and so on.

- *The point person:* If it's your physician's nurse who takes the calls, be sure to say hello. Matching a name with a (smiling) face helps make subsequent encounters easier. Always remember that if you're treated well by someone in particular, be sure to tell your physician. And a small token of your appreciation such as a fresh plate of cookies will go a long way in creating a great relationship with your physician's staff members and paving the way for effortless care the next time you really need something.

WHEN TO INSIST ON A SPECIALIST

Whether your pediatrician seeks a referral may depend on the type of practice she maintains. In this era of managed care and tight profit margins, physicians have to see more and more patients to maintain their bottom line. As we've all probably experienced, the patient pays the price, getting shorter visits and quicker decisions. In some high-volume practices your physician may choose to refer to a specialist at the earliest sign of a problem. Some find it easier to try to get help as soon as possible—much like a business that likes to outsource the work that it can't do profitably. In this case, your physician may have a relationship with a specialist that is based on previous success.

Some practices, on the other hand, are more old-fashioned in their approach and may try everything before involving a

REFLUX REALITY

What Your Physician May Be Thinking

I'm always surprised when parents tell me that they want to do something other than what I've prescribed. After all, they have come to me to solve a problem, and I have offered a solution.

I recently cared for a 2-month-old infant with severe acid reflux and difficulty feeding. After a thorough evaluation, I talked with the family and suggested treating the reflux with one of our most frequently used medications. The mother, in this case, had investigated reflux on the Internet. Prepared for my recommendation, she expressed concern for a rare side effect called permanent tardive dyskinesia. I did my best to allay her fears, but the experience and authority of a chat-room stranger took precedence in her mind. The final compromise was to give the baby an alternate medication, in this case an antacid. At the follow-up visit 3 weeks later, I found that the baby still had moderate heartburn symptoms and poor weight gain. Revisiting my original treatment plan, I was able to help the mother to understand that the small risk of side effects in this case had to be balanced with the benefits the medication could provide. Achieving this delicate balance of risk and benefit requires excellent clinical judgment, years of experience, consideration of the complicated social circumstances that every patient brings to the exam room, and, not least, personal knowledge of the patient. For better or worse, none of this can be found on the Internet.

The Internet has indelibly changed the physician–patient relationship. The monopoly on information that physicians once held no longer exists. Physicians now answer to patients almost as much as we inform patients. We modify what parents have already learned on their own and help them shape decisions that they're comfortable with.

I'll leave you to decide whether all of this change is a good thing. Either way, patients have more power than ever in controlling their medical destiny and that of their children. But with that power comes responsibility. Patients have a responsibility to understand the limits of their knowledge despite their limitless access to information. Although some physicians have done their part to erode the confidence of their patients over the past generation, health care consumers with unrestricted access to information are doing their part to redefine the physician–patient relationship in this generation.

pediatric gastroenterologist. In this more traditional primary care model, you will need to decide whether you're comfortable with the results you're getting from your physician. If your physician has a plan of treatment, it's best to stick it out. But if your physician's plan involves formula roulette and erratic changes in treatment every week while your baby continues to do poorly, it may be time to ask for a referral or seek one yourself. Many of my self-referrals come from parents who don't feel that enough is being done for their baby.

Most babies with reflux will never need to see the inside of a gastroenterologist's office, but every pediatrician and parent is within their rights to look for help when uncomfortable. In most cases, the decision to seek the input of a pediatric gastroenterologist will depend on you, your baby, and your pediatrician, or, more important, on how all three parties feel about one another.

Knowing When You Absolutely Need
to See a Pediatric Gastroenterologist

There are some absolute indications for getting some extra input when your baby has reflux:

- *Sick babies who aren't getting better:* Sometimes babies are just plain sick and their condition necessitates more advanced input for managing their problem. If your baby has any of the complications of reflux detailed in Chapter 4 ("Recognizing the Sick Baby: When It's More Than Just the Spits") and initial attempts by your physician have been unsuccessful, your baby should be under the care of a pediatric gastroenterologist. The complications involving breathing and growth concern us the most. Good pediatricians are experts in identifying sick babies.
- *Reflux that doesn't go away:* If your baby has made it to age 18 months or beyond and still has symptoms of reflux, you may want to get a second look. Your pediatrician may refer you earlier, however.
- *Reflux that doesn't follow the book:* If your baby's symptoms don't follow what one would expect from a baby with reflux, it might be worth getting a second opinion for your child. For example, remember that symptoms of reflux in infancy commonly begin in the first 2 to 4 months of life. Reflux that begins late in infancy is unusual and should raise suspicions that something else may be going on with your baby. Deviations from what we know and expect of infant reflux should raise eyebrows.
- *When things are unclear:* If there are potential concerns about your baby's condition, it's better to be safe than

sorry. A one-time visit doesn't commit you to a lifelong relationship with a second physician.

What Will a Pediatric Gastroenterologist Do Differently from a Pediatrician?

What might I expect when I take my child to a pediatric gastroenterologist? What can he do that my pediatrician can't? Pediatric gastroenterologists are pediatricians who spend an extra 3 years after their pediatric residency learning about childhood intestinal disease. They are required to first become board-certified pediatricians before qualifying for board certification in gastroenterology. All this extra training and extra experience make pediatric gastroenterologists more adept at identifying reflux complications and risk factors for complications. They're going to know when to take the next step as far as invasive testing. And they're going to be more adept at interpreting the variations in test results.

From the treatment side, you might expect a greater level of comfort with the various medications and formulas available to treat babies with intestinal problems. Truth be told, most of the children who see me in consultation have been headed in the right direction by their pediatrician but just need their medicines and nutritional regimen tweaked.

Pediatric Gastroenterologists—Private and Public

Pediatric gastroenterologists typically practice in one of two settings: academic and private. Academic pediatric gastroenterologists typically work in large children's hospitals and medical centers. Their responsibilities beyond caring for children involve research and teaching. Private gastroenterologists are in business for themselves or some other large specialty practice. Their day-to-day activities typically involve only caring for kids.

So what difference does this make for you and your baby? In a perfect world, it shouldn't make any difference. But reality dictates that there are differences in the care that your child may receive in an academic versus a private setting. Private offices, because they're small and independent, may offer a more intimate experience. But if your child has a rare problem that involves the intestinal tract, you may find greater expertise in a larger academically oriented children's hospital. In either case, your child's care will ultimately depend on the experience and skill of your physician. That can vary tremendously independent of where you seek care.

Kids with Tummy Aches Looking for Help— a Seller's Market

All this talk about picking the type of practice you want for your baby is hypothetical because pediatric gastroenterologists are few and far between. In fact, if you live in a small to midsize city, you may have only one or two pediatric gastroenterologists to choose from, and that's if you're lucky. In some instances you may be forced to drive 3 to 4 hours to the nearest big city for help.

But how can that be? This is America, land of the ever-discriminating patient-consumer. If we don't like our physicians, we fire them. But because of a workforce report issued by the NASPGHAN in 1997 predicting a future glut of pediatric gastroenterologists, some training programs subsequently closed down and the pipeline of freshly minted tummy docs slowed to a gentle trickle. In 2004, only 24 pediatric gastroenterologists completed their training, and in that year there were more than 170 positions unfilled in that field. The field is recovering, but it will take some years to produce the physicians needed to fill the demands of an ever-expanding population and the vacancies left by retiring specialists.

Finding a Qualified Pediatric Gastroenterologist

Because there aren't enough of us to go around, you may not have the option of being picky when selecting a physician for your baby. Your best resource will, of course, be your pediatrician, who should be able to point you in the right direction. If your pediatrician doesn't want to refer you, you can consider placing a call to another pediatric practice in town and explain your situation—just ask who they use for pediatric GI referrals. Most offices disclose this information without a hitch. If there are other pediatric specialists in your area, they may serve as a resource for you as well. Allergists, pediatric surgeons, and ear, nose, and throat specialists often work closely with pediatric stomach specialists. But if you think your baby needs more help and your pediatrician isn't providing it or willing to outsource it, it may be time to look for another physician.

You can also identify a pediatric gastroenterologist in your area by going to www.naspghan.org, the address of the website for the North American Society of Pediatric Gastroenterology, Hepatology, and Nutrition, which has a physician-locator option that you can use. While a physician's membership in NASPGHAN doesn't necessarily mean that you will like him or that he'll give you what you need, it's a good place to start.

WHAT KIND OF INFORMATION WILL THE PEDIATRIC GASTROENTEROLOGIST NEED TO EVALUATE YOUR CHILD?

To make the most of your visit, it helps to do your homework. Here's some information you may want to have handy on the day of your visit:

- *Progress so far:* What medications has your baby been taking? What are the dosages, how long were they used, and what was the response?
- *Patterns of feeding:* How much does your baby take at a feed, how long does it take, and what does she look like when she's taking it? Be sure to know the daily volume that your baby takes in. Remember that feeding tells us a lot about a baby's reflux.
- *Patterns of irritability and spitting:* When do your baby's symptoms appear to be worse? Are there things that seem to make her symptoms better, such as positioning? When does your baby vomit in reference to feeding and what does it look like?
- *Patterns of pooping:* How often does your baby poop, what does it look like, and how does she look when she's doing it? Remember that the presence of blood and mucus can be indicative of milk protein allergy. Sometimes fussy behavior is the only sign.
- *Records:* While you may be inclined to tote every scrap of your child's medical record to your specialist visit, it may be overkill. Check with the physician's office to see what exactly is needed. In many cases the only helpful information is blood work, X-ray results, and growth curves. Growth charts are critical if weight gain has been a problem.

Absolutely Never Let a Gastroenterologist
Who Specializes in Adults Treat Your Child

In the same way that you'd never trust your accountant to replace the brakes on your minivan, you should never ask a gastroenterologist who specializes in adults to look after your kids. Children are not small adults. The way that their diseases appear, the way they metabolize reflux medication, their reflux complications, and so many other issues particular to children make adult-trained specialists a bad choice for GI care in kids. Because of the risks associated with practicing outside of one's specialty, malpractice insurance carriers have all but mandated that adult-trained gastroenterologists not treat children. But if you have good insurance or are willing to pay cash, you may find someone who's willing to roll the dice and take a crack at your child. Just say no.

What Does a Lack of Pediatric Gastroenterologists
Mean for Your Baby?

What this all means is that you may have a harder time getting to see a specialist should your baby need one. Some pediatricians know they lack the backup that they would like to have and are often forced to handle things on their own. You as a parent have to be vigilant about your baby's care. Be informed and ask all the questions you need to ensure that your baby gets the treatment she needs.

10

REFLUX BEYOND INFANCY

What to Do When the Reflux That's Supposed to Have Gone Away Hasn't

Okay, so your baby is 14 months old and she's still spitting up throughout the day. It's not supposed to be this way. All the books say that this problem should be gone by now, and even your pediatrician is starting to look as uncomfortable as a long drive from the beach in a wet bathing suit. So what do you do when reflux just won't go away?

The first thing that you need to do is adjust your expectations. A child's first birthday can be a tricky time for the parent of a refluxing child because popular opinion says that this is when all of the problems go away. In most infants the symptoms of reflux resolve somewhere between 4 and 12 months of age. It's during this time that the immature intestinal tract matures and begins to do what it is supposed to do. The poor emptying of the stomach and the frequent relaxations of the "valve" above the stomach resolve, and food begins to stay put. At 6 months of age, babies begin to spend more time vertical, which puts gravity on their side. The addition of solid food may help as well.

Realistically, however, reflux can linger well beyond a baby's first birthday. The statistics of who does what when aren't perfectly clear because the range of symptoms that babies can have is so broad. Remember that among babies who spit up, 95% stop spitting up by 1 year of age. In babies sicker during infancy, there's evidence to suggest that 80% have resolved their reflux by 12 to 24 months of age. *Bottom line:* It's safe to say, on the basis of limited epidemiologic data and vast clinical experience, that sick or not, most babies outgrow their reflux by 1 year of age. In some, it lingers until their second birthday, and in a very small number, reflux continues into late toddlerhood and the early school years.

But is that the end of the story? Maybe not. There are some recent studies from Australia that looked at babies with acid reflux and monitored them through their school years. It seems that despite what we have always thought was a baby problem may have implications for older children. Children between 8 and 11 years of age who had reflux as infants were nearly five times more likely to experience regular heartburn than other children. Children who had reflux as babies seem to be about three times more likely to have regular vomiting than their peers, and their overall risk of some type of reflux symptom is 2.3 times greater. While more follow-up work needs to be done, particularly with those babies who go on to have symptoms as children, these data suggest that infant reflux may be a foreshadowing of things to come.

THERE ARE TWO TYPES OF REFLUX: BABY AND ADULT

Up to this point, I've suggested that reflux is something that always goes away. In most cases, it does. However, some toddlers

> **REFLUX REALITY**
>
> *"Reflux Always Goes Away"*
>
> False. Though most babies grow out of their reflux, a small percentage will continue through toddlerhood and into childhood with symptoms of GER.

are like big babies when it comes to spitting up and just seem to need a little more time. Early reflux and everything we've talked about so far falls into what we call *infant reflux*. That is the self-limited, largely harmless but often annoying speed bump of intestinal motility that makes babies spit up, scream, and sputter. And though it may not always go away as quickly as we'd like, it's rare that it doesn't go away at all.

Those of you with reflux or with older children with reflux can probably appreciate that your reflux is very different from your baby's. Reflux that begins in childhood or adulthood is referred to as *adult reflux*. As I've suggested, a tiny number of infants never let go of their reflux and grow into childhood with symptoms that seem to persist. This infant reflux becomes adult reflux when it continues beyond toddlerhood and shows no sign of stopping. But despite what may look like two different conditions, adult reflux and infant reflux are effectively the same thing: a motility disorder that causes gastric contents to wash up where they don't belong, wreaking havoc along the way. The difference between the two boils down to

- *Chronicity:* Adult reflux tends to be chronic, or at least relapsing in nature. It is estimated that among children and adults with reflux, about 50% will require some type of long-term therapy. Infant reflux is typically self-limited.

- *Expression of symptoms:* One of the obvious differences between your 10-week-old and your 10-year-old is their capacity for telling you what's going on. Older children and adults can describe chest pain, painful regurgitation, difficulty swallowing, and many of the other symptoms that characterize adult reflux disease.

- *Long-term effects:* Beyond just describing their symptoms, what we see in children and adults can be more involved. The damage from reflux and its secondary complications can create different symptoms and sensations that create the appearance of a different problem.

Why Does Reflux Hang On in Some Toddlers?

So what is it about some children and adults that causes them to have reflux? This isn't exactly known, although the roots of adult reflux are no different than for infant reflux. We know that the poor motility of infancy improves with time and maturity, and this explains why most infant reflux goes away. Adult reflux stems from similar problems of poor motility, incompetent LES function, and perhaps issues with excessive acid. The difference is that it never quite goes away. In families where there is a strong history of severe reflux, there may be issues with the nerves or the way nerves talk to one another that creates the milieu for reflux disease and its complications. The same holds true for toddlers. Some children are genetically marked for reflux and it never quite resolves itself.

The Fuzzy Line Between Infant and Adult Reflux

So how can you know if your toddler is one of these babies des-
tined to have reflux over the coming years? From personal experience, I can tell you that it's very difficult. The signs or
symptoms in a toddler that predict whether reflux will ultimately resolve are unknown. In the real world, we simply treat
babies to control their symptoms, monitor them for complications, and hope that it goes away.

There's no reason to be concerned if your child continues to
have symptoms of reflux at ages 12 to 24 months. But with that
said, if your child still has symptoms by 18 months of age and
she hasn't yet seen a pediatric gastroenterologist, you should
probably set up an appointment. Gastroenterologists may not
do too much differently from what your pediatrician has done,
but they have a keen eye for some of the subtle signs of brew-
ing complications.

Beyond 24 months of age, the odds are beginning to work
against you that this is a self-limited problem of infancy. It's
not that it can't go away, it's just that the developmental problems that create infant reflux should have sorted themselves
out by this point. Even so, I must say that I have cared for many
toddlers beyond their second birthday whose reflux has spontaneously resolved after a period of supportive medical care. I've
also seen many who grow into their early school years requiring close follow-up, further evaluation, and treatment.

Sometimes We Like to Wait Until Children Can Talk to Us

Older children are better than younger ones at telling us about
their reflux. Sometimes the subtle symptoms of poor sleeping

or poor eating that seem to respond to treatment make themselves clear as children get beyond their third or fourth birthday and can begin to vocalize their symptoms.

This is particularly important in the toddler with chronic lung symptoms that we think are related to acid reflux. When reflux symptoms are present and a child's breathing symptoms don't respond to asthma therapy, treatment for reflux certainly is indicated. When this doesn't help matters and we're still concerned about reflux disease, it may be time to consider anti-reflux surgery. Sometimes patience will allow either the reflux to improve or the child to mature to a point where she can tell us what she's feeling. Remember that diagnostic techniques such as pH probes aren't always perfect at picking up the connection between reflux and its role in lung disease. A child's report of chronic throat burning or chest pain may help seal the deal by proving that reflux is a problem despite therapy with the best reflux medications.

The Toddler Who Can't Be Weaned from a Proton Pump Inhibitor

One of the most challenging and frustrating scenarios is the toddler or preschooler with reflux who is absolutely symptom free when taking an acid suppressant but develops bothersome symptoms when his therapy is discontinued. For example, he takes a PPI every day, but when he stops, symptoms of nighttime awakening and throat-clearing reappear.

The situation is challenging because the problem doesn't appear to be going away, but then again, the child doesn't seem that sick. In many cases like this, endoscopy shows no significant esophageal damage because the child has been treated.

This is the scenario of the child dependent on her acid suppression and unable to do without it.

In these cases, you may have to come to terms with the fact that your child has a chronic condition and that the effects of unchecked reflux may be greater than any known effects of the medications. It's important to understand in a toddler that there is still a chance that the condition could resolve on its own. In the older child, this may be something that you will have to live with. Periodic "holidays" from medication will confirm whether ongoing treatment is still needed. This is certainly a situation that requires close monitoring by a pediatric gastroenterologist.

As a child grows, her ability to relate the extent of her symptoms to us may allow us to make more educated decisions about therapy. Some families, for example, whose children are clearly dependent on acid suppression for chronic reflux disease choose to consider surgery as an alternative to long-term medical therapy.

Reflux Medications Aren't Good-Luck Charms

Sometimes parents have a hard time letting go of their child's reflux medication. With the indelible memory of sleepless, miserable nights, it's easy to understand how some would never want to experience the bad times again. But such fears can create something of a dependency for parents. They come to see their child's medication as pivotal to their ongoing symptom-free success. But in reality, the reflux may not exist anymore and they're just unwilling to risk stopping treatment. Reflux medications are not good-luck charms to hang on to for security.

WHEN YOUR CHILD GETS A PINK SLIP FROM DAY CARE

Vomiting or regurgitation is often a one-way ticket home for tots in day care. This typically arises because of policies put in place to prevent tummy bugs from being passed around. If your day care puts up a battle about your child's reflux, the staff members may need nothing more than a little education. Talk to your physician about providing a brief letter explaining your child's condition.

Conversely, there's a tendency for parents to become hyper-vigilant when medications are discontinued. The slightest burp or the first episode of awakening is met with panic and they make a beeline for the medicine cabinet. If your doctor has recommended a trial without medications, keep an open mind and give your child time to show herself as truly having symptoms requiring treatment. Try to allow your child a period of 2 to 3 weeks so that a symptom can be reproduced and definitely associated with the discontinuation of the medication.

SYMPTOMS THAT SUGGEST REFLUX IN TODDLERS AND YOUNG CHILDREN

One trap that parents can fall into is the assumption that if their baby's spitting up has resolved, so has the reflux. But remember that some of our sickest babies with reflux never spit up a day in their lives, and so it goes for the older set. The absence of stuff coming out of the mouth says little about what a child may be experiencing in the throat and below.

REFLUX THERAPY IN TODDLERS VERSUS INFANTS

When it comes to the treatment of reflux, toddlers might just as well be big babies. The treatment doesn't vary much. But here are some things that you may notice:

- *Expect more therapy with antacids alone.* Prokinetic medications such as metoclopramide and bethanechol are less likely to be used because of their marginal efficacy compounded by the practical difficulty of dispensing a medication four times daily to a 2-year-old.
- *Expect more comfort with newer medications.* Some physicians who are skeptical of the safety of PPI in babies may come around to the idea after the child's first birthday.
- *Expect input from a pediatric gastroenterolgist.* If your child has symptoms of reflux at age 18 months, you might find your physician making a referral for help.

What are the common signs and symptoms of GER in children beyond infancy?

Poor Sleeping

If you've encountered it firsthand or read any of the popular parenting guides, you're probably aware that beginning late in the first year, children often awaken in the middle of the night only to find themselves alone in the dark. Their immediate natural response in many cases is to cry for help, which typi-

TALES FROM THE CRIB

Twenty-Month-Old with Reflux That Doesn't Seem to Be Going Away

Presentation

Diego is a 20-month-old with GER that just keeps hanging on. His early months were marked with chronic spitting, poor feeding, and irritability. After 6 months of age and appropriate treatment, he was less irritable, but he never stopped spitting up.

Currently, Diego urps up one or two times most days and occasionally vomits. His vomiting has been known to occur 2 to 3 hours after meals and seems to be most noticeable after eating fast food. This has created difficulties when eating out or in playgroups. His day care has sent him home on two occasions with concerns that he had something contagious. Without acid suppression, Diego eats less and experiences frequent nighttime awakening. When given a once-a-day PPI, his symptoms of poor eating and poor sleeping decreased, although little has helped his regurgitation and vomiting. Prokinetic medications, including bethanechol, metoclopramide, and erythromycin, have been tried but with little to no improvement. His evaluation has included an upper GI series and basic blood work, the results of which have been unremarkable. Growth has never been an issue, and there have been no signs or symptoms attributable to his lungs.

With every month that passes, his parents become more concerned because they thought the reflux was supposed to be gone by now. Everything they read tells them that this isn't normal. His pediatrician has asked the family to be patient, although the family senses that even he is beginning to question why Diego is doing what he's doing.

Analysis

Diego's reflux of infancy hasn't gone away, and it's unclear when and if it will. It doesn't seem that bad, but then again, urping and vomiting at this age isn't normal. Pediatricians are often at a loss when reflux doesn't do what it's supposed to do (disappear after 1 year). But the truth is that pediatric gastroenterologists find themselves similarly stuck regarding the child who's not quite out of infant reflux but yet not quite far enough along to be declared as having a chronic problem. Welcome to the no-man's-land of toddler reflux.

Is there anything else that we might do to evaluate a child like this? Many pediatric gastroenterologists would consider an upper endoscopy at this point. This would eliminate the possibility of an allergic or inflammatory condition causing his spitting up and vomiting. But such an effective response to PPI might make this less likely, however. The odds of his having any ongoing damage to the esophagus from reflux while receiving such excellent therapy is unlikely. He had an upper GI series, so we can feel comfortable knowing that there's nothing awry with his anatomy. A pH probe is unlikely to change what we're going to do at this point, because Diego appears to have reflux responsive to medications. Some pediatric gastroenterologists might be interested in determining how much reflux Diego has, and in this case a pH probe would be helpful. But again, it's unlikely to change the management of his disease in the short term.

The fact that prokinetic agents aren't helping in this case isn't surprising. Prokinetic agents such as metoclopramide and bethanechol are not proven to be of much help in reflux, although reflux in some babies may respond. The response in toddlers like Diego tends to be more predictably unreliable.

With regard to what we should do at this point, Diego hasn't suffered any consequences from his reflux, so it's hard to build an argument for being very aggressive. At this point his reflux seems to be nothing more than a nuisance. While it's not a satisfying plan for anyone involved, I would recommend in this case continuing to treat with acid suppressants. I would continue to support the family, suggest tile floors for their house, and continue to monitor for complications of reflux.

Though with the passage of each month the odds of spontaneous resolution dwindle, there is hope that the reflux will decrease. In cases such as this, I will monitor Diego to the point where he is developmentally better able to describe his symptoms. Then, should he continue to have chronic symptoms, I would discuss with the family options for long-term management of his reflux, including use of acid suppressants and even fundoplication.

cally results in Mom or Dad making the fifty-yard dash to the nursery. When they see your face, the anxiety of their isolation is resolved and their disposition turns quickly for the better. One of the tricky issues that we frequently face in this age group is discriminating reflux awakening from behavioral nighttime awakening.

Sorting this issue out can be difficult. Because reflux likes to rear its ugly head at night, sleep disturbance may be one of the only signs that your child is dealing with reflux. In late infancy and toddlerhood, this may amount to awakening in the night screaming and crying. While it can be difficult to identify the signs, children awakening with reflux usually do so because they're hurting. When you greet them, you may find them arching, turning their head, clearing their throat, grabbing or pulling at their chest or neck, hitting their ears, or indicating in some other way that they're uncomfortable. One helpful indicator of reflux pain may be the presence of ongoing screaming despite your being there. Remember that esophageal burning and throat pain don't disappear with your appearance. With behavioral nighttime awakening, however, you are more apt to see your child settle almost immediately when you arrive.

But not every child with nocturnal reflux wakes up and cries. Other common signs of reflux in children include chronic nighttime cough, throat clearing, restlessness, and morning hoarseness. The older children are, the better they become at telling us what's going on or seeking help on their own. Some children will seek water at night; others may find comfort with a second pillow.

Chronic Hoarseness

As soon as kids have the capacity to make noise, they have the ability to tell us that they may have reflux. While less frequent in infancy, changes in voice quality with crying can come with reflux. More often, hoarseness is an indicator of chronic reflux in older children. Hoarseness arises from the subtle change in elasticity of the vocal cords that often comes from chronic acid exposure. As we discussed previously under "Poor Sleeping," hoarseness that improves a couple of hours after awakening can be an indicator of nighttime reflux.

If your child is chronically hoarse, her first stop may be to see an ear, nose, and throat specialist. That evaluation will usually involve looking at the throat and vocal cords with a tiny fiber-optic camera. One of the most common findings in children with hoarseness due to reflux is *vocal cord nodules*, or small reactive bumps or blebs on the vocal cords themselves. They often go away with reflux therapy but sometimes require speech therapy.

Eating Problems

The capacity to handle and accept lumpy, bumpy textures in foods is an important skill acquired late in the first year of life. You may remember that back in Chapter 4 ("Recognizing the Sick Baby: When It's More Than Just the Spits") we discussed oral sensory aversion, one of the bothersome complications of unchecked reflux. If it goes untreated, difficulties with solid textures will follow children well into toddlerhood and beyond.

Beyond the obvious choking and gagging that occurs with sensory aversion, kids can have other eating-related problems associated with acid reflux:

- *Difficulty swallowing (dysphagia):* Children with esophageal inflammation commonly experience difficulty swallowing dense foods such as meat and doughy breads. This is because the esophagus is a very sensitive and intricate organ that squeezes and pushes in a very methodic way, depending on what goes into it. And when it's unhappy, it doesn't do its job of squeezing. It's no different from an inflamed knee or elbow that can't bend in the way that it's supposed to.

- *Picky eating:* Over time, children with reflux esophagitis can become conditioned to the fact that when they eat, they'll hurt. When no effort is made to look for occult, or hidden, symptoms of reflux, this conditioned behavior is often perceived as picky eating. GER should always be on your physician's short list of possibilities when you report poor eating in your child.

- *Burning with acidic foods:* An irritated esophagus is sensitive to what touches it, much like a skinned knee or a paper cut that stings when touched by the wrong stuff. The most common perpetrators are acidic foods such as citrus juice and tomato-based foods. And children get quite adept at avoiding acidic foods, even when they don't know why.

Heartburn

If you want to know if your child has reflux, just ask. I never cease to be amazed at the number of children I see in consultation who have never been asked about reflux. Missing reflux in babies is one thing that I can forgive, but missing a diagnosis because we didn't ask is something that's harder to overlook. And you can do it yourself. My favorite screen for symptomatic reflux in children older than 5 years of age or so is the following question: "Have you ever had that sour taste in your mouth like you're going to throw up but you don't throw up? Instead you just swallow it?"

Now, in my line of work, I've become quite accustomed to judging the response that I get from school-age kids when asked that question. Children who suffer with chronic reflux will immediately light up and recognize your description as something that they've felt for some time. In most cases, they never knew that it was something that they should complain about. Many think that the sensation of reflux is just normal. Parents who think they know everything about their kids are often just as surprised as their children are when they learn about what they're suffering with every day.

Those children who look puzzled, have to think, or immediately answer no generally aren't experiencing much of what we consider reflux while awake. Reflux, of course, can occur when we're not aware of it, such as at night when sleeping.

Answers to this quizzing about stuff in the throat typically begin to be reliable after about age 5 years, or perhaps age 4 in a bright, engaging child. Younger children will tell us about their heartburn in one way or another. This can involve throat-grabbing, lip-smacking, grimacing, or "bitter beer face" (a description that came from a father). Self-gagging is another strange sign of reflux. Apparently, the sensation of gagging offers some relief when reflux is stuck somewhere betwixt and between ("either go back down or come up!").

Chest Pain

The term *heartburn* refers to the fiery sensation under the sternum that we adults often experience with reflux. In some children, old-fashioned heartburn is the indicator of reflux. Most often described as pain or heaviness on the chest, heartburn in children can raise concerns about a heart attack, especially when you ask an adult specialist to evaluate your child. Sometimes the sensation of tightness in the chest that comes with exercise can lead pediatricians down the asthma path. And for

IF YOU DON'T ASK, THEY WON'T TELL

If you want to know if your child has reflux, it's sometimes simply a matter of asking. Very often children become accustomed to the symptoms of reflux that they experience day in and day out. If you don't ask, you may never know.

good reason, the symptoms can look remarkably alike. Typically, ongoing symptoms of pain with appropriate asthma medications and a physical exam without wheezing will get a good physician on the right track.

Abdominal Pain

As adults we all know that reflux gives us the sensation of heartburn—a heavy, dull pain in the chest often associated with throat burning and regurgitation. While heartburn can masquerade as things such as a heart attack in old folks, its presentation is pretty predictable. With kids, it isn't always so straightforward. It all goes back to a child's developmental ability to describe and localize symptoms. Early school-age children lack the capacity to describe their symptoms in the most precise words. And when it comes to discomfort anywhere from the chest to the groin, they will point to the belly button. After about 10 years of age, kids become better able to tell us where their pain is and use good descriptive terms to explain their experience. In toddlers and young school-age kids, we have to look beyond the simple report of pain and inquire about wet burps, pain after and during eating, throat-clearing,

---

HOW YOUR CHILD MAY DESCRIBE REFLUX

- Sour burps
- Hot burps
- Sore throat
- Fiery burps

- Burning in the throat
- Spicy throat
- Fire in the throat

---

and nausea—symptoms that may lead us to suspect reflux as a possible perpetrator.

A study not so long ago looked at the characteristics of children presenting to the emergency room with GER. Know what the leading complaint was? Bellyache. Falling not that far behind were asthmalike symptoms, chest pain, and regurgitation. This wasn't necessarily an earth-shaking study, but it raised the important point that reflux in children may not always appear as straightforward as reflux in adults.

WHEN REFLUX APPEARS OVERNIGHT IN YOUR CHILD

Sometimes reflux seems to appear overnight in children. A child who was previously well begins reporting regurgitation and sore throat with chest pain. How can this be when we've painted the picture of reflux as a chronic problem? Children can develop reflux acutely.

Viral Infections

The same problems with motility that predispose children to chronic reflux can appear out of the blue after a stomach in-

---

CAN REFLUX BE INFECTIOUS?

Could your child's reflux be fixed with antibiotics? Possibly. There's a bacteria called *Helicobacter pylori* that likes to take up residence in the lining of the stomach, where it can predispose people to gastritis and ulcers. In fact, most ulcers in adults are caused by this pesky bug. When children are infected, they'll complain of bellyache, nausea, and sometimes reflux symptoms. A blood test exists to look for this infection, but it isn't always reliable. The presence of this infection is best established with endoscopy or with a test called a urea breath test.

---

jury. One of the most common causes of acute injury that can create reflux is a GI bug. The simple irritation that comes with a garden-variety intestinal virus can cause a child to complain of reflux symptoms. When unhappy or inflamed, the tummy may not squeeze and empty the way that it should, just as in the baby with milk protein allergy. Children in this situation often report reflux symptoms and even pain after eating. Fortunately, this tends to be a self-limited type of reflux that goes away when the irritation goes away. This can sometimes take 4 to 8 weeks from the onset of symptoms and may be helped with the use of acid suppressants as prescribed by your physician.

Medication Gastritis

Medications are another common cause of "acute reflux" in children. The child taking numerous medications for, say, asthma or seizures can sometimes develop chemical gastritis with reflux and tummy pain. Nonsteroidal anti-inflammatory drugs such as ibuprofen can cause stomach inflammation and reflux. Alteration in medications and dosing typically do the trick, but sometimes traditional treatment is necessary.

Pizza Parties, Pajama Parties, and Other Things That Make Us Go Urp in the Night

And finally, as with adults, dietary indiscretions play a role in childhood reflux. A big night on the town with pepperoni pizza, carbonated drinks, and ice cream sundaes doesn't help any child's upper intestinal motility. Too much of the wrong thing can predispose your child to a sudden case of the urps.

WHAT (OR WHAT NOT) TO FEED THE REFLUXING TODDLER

Speaking of pizza and too much of a good thing, are there things that can be done with a child's diet to decrease reflux? Perhaps. Because we've been dealing with reflux in infancy up until now, we haven't had a whole lot of dietary leverage at hand. Now that we're into the toddler and preschool years, we're dealing with a variety of foods that can have an impact on a child's intestinal physiology. But seizing control may be easier said than done.

One of the glaring challenges that we face every day with toddlers and preschoolers is the natural difficulty in influencing a child's intake. As adults, we can avoid certain kinds of foods or increase our intake of other foods because we understand what's at stake (usually). Two-year-olds have a harder time hearing the voice of reason. Two-year-olds eat what they want, when they feel like it, with absolutely no regard for whether you've worked hard to prepare it or how good it may be for them. A toddler's drive to eat is based solely on metabolism, tempered by a fickle view of their immediate environment. Dietary manipulation as a primary approach to controlling childhood reflux before 4 or 5 years of age tends to work well in textbooks but not always in the real world.

With that disclaimer on record, there are some things that you can try to leave out of the grocery cart. Remember that if it isn't in the pantry, there's no way they can eat it!

Six Dietary Tips That May Help the Child with Reflux

- *Watch the transition to whole milk.* Physicians recommend that children who are bottle-fed or who choose to wean from breast milk transition to whole milk at 1 year of age. The preference for whole milk, as opposed to skim or 2%, stems from the fact that it offers more calories for toddlers who are notoriously picky. You may notice a flare in your child's reflux symptoms after the transition to whole milk. The solute load, or "stuff," in whole milk (protein, sodium, potassium) is greater than in breast milk or formula. This can add up to slower digestion and potentially more reflux. If your child eats well and her reflux seems to be worse after switching to whole milk, you can talk to your physician about considering a trial of lower-fat milk. Another option is the use of a toddler formula.
- *Avoid carbonated beverages.* Fizz that goes down must come up. Soda, which contains too many empty calories, should have no role in your child's diet, with or without reflux. Choose water or diluted 100% juices.

- *Avoid fast food.* Fast food tends to be high in fat, which slows gastric emptying and contributes to reflux.
- *Avoid chocolate.* Chocolate has a tendency to decrease the tightness of the LES, the valve that keeps your child from refluxing. And independent of this unique physiologic phenomenon, most chocolate rides along with other heavy ingredients such as saturated fat and sugar, things that won't help GERD.
- *Use low-acid foods.* Foods that are citrus- or tomato-based are more apt to make your child hurt, especially if he has esophagitis. Simple avoidance is the best policy. Some orange juice manufacturers are now making low-acid products for the ever-growing reflux market.
- *Don't let your child eat within 3 hours of bedtime.* Give your child's tummy time to work before making it fight gravity. Avoid letting him snack before bed.

Remember: Diet Rarely Fixes Chronic Pediatric Reflux

With the exception of the child suffering with acute post-viral reflux, dietary changes are rarely ever enough to keep a refluxing child medication free. While that's no excuse for not making sensible food choices, keep your expectations realistic.

WORST-CASE SCENARIO—WHEN REFLUX GOES BAD

In Chapter 4 ("Recognizing the Sick Baby: When It's More Than Just the Spits") we discussed the things that we worry about in refluxing babies. The concerns in toddlers and older children change a little bit because as children continue to experience reflux over the months, the odds of damage from reflux increases. My intention in discussing the common complications of reflux is not to make parents nervous and on edge about their children. I simply want to make it clear that despite the general belief that reflux is merely a laundry problem, it must be monitored to ensure that it doesn't become a true medical problem.

Heartburn Gone Wild—
Esophagitis and Esophageal Stricture

We already know that reflux can irritate the esophagus to the point of making a baby scream inconsolably. I mentioned in Chapter 4 ("Recognizing the Sick Baby: When It's More Than Just the Spits") that most babies, despite how loudly they may scream, are NERD babies; they have *nonerosive reflux disease*. They may scream as though they have open sores in their esophagus, but our experience tells us that it's typically irritation that hasn't reached the point of deep erosions.

Months of acid exposure in the esophagus, however, can create damage referred to as *erosive esophagitis*, a serious problem. Through an endoscope, the esophagus in a child with reflux esophagitis can be seen to be pale and swollen with furrows or lines where the acid has done its damage. The scary thing is that it can be difficult to predict which children will develop erosive esophagitis. We get suspicious, however, when faced with a young child with chronic reflux, difficulty swallowing, and chronic pain after eating. The presence of blood in the stool or in vomit will sometimes offer a clue, but oftentimes vomiting isn't even a symptom.

Among children who fail to complain, or worse, fail to have their complaints evaluated, unchecked reflux esophagitis can have irreversible consequences. Over time, inflammation of the esophagus lining can develop into scar tissue in the most involved areas. As this evolves, the esophagus develops a nondistensible hourglass narrowing referred to as a *stricture*. Once this occurs, the damage from reflux can't be reversed and a child is then committed to a lifetime of periodic stretching, or dilation, of the stricture to be able to eat. During esophageal dilation, a pediatric gastroenterologist places a balloon through an endoscope at the site of narrowing and inflates it. The scar stretches, only to shrink down again as the months pass. Children with esophageal stricture are typically considered candidates for fundoplication to prevent further reflux damage in an already badly inflamed esophagus.

Chronic Asthma

One of the most hotly debated arguments in pediatric medicine is the relationship between chronic asthma and GER. The symptoms of reflux are common in children with asthma, but establishing a cause–effect relationship can be difficult. According to the most recent figures from the National Center for Health Statistics, asthma affects an estimated 6.1 million children in the United States. Furthermore, about 60% of children with chronic asthma have abnormal findings on pH probe tests. But even among those asthmatic children with proven reflux, only about 50% have the symptoms that we typically associate with reflux. We have to remain openminded about the potential for reflux when faced with a wheezing child even when the story doesn't suggest it.

Whom do we test and whom do we treat? A lot of this will

depend on whose office you wind up in. Different folks have different ideas about this reflux–asthma connection, and experience can vary tremendously. Some allergists and pulmonary specialists are aware of the role of reflux in their world; others are a little behind the times. If your asthma specialist isn't at least thinking about it, you should ask why or consider looking elsewhere.

Most children with symptoms of heartburn or regurgitation with their asthma could benefit from at least a trial of antireflux medication. Clinical studies show that among asthmatic children with reflux, more than 60% of those treated for reflux had improvement in their asthma symptoms as well as a reduction in the use of bronchodilator medications. The secret is that children have to be treated with appropriate doses of acid suppression for a long enough period of time. Three months of consistent therapy would be considered the minimum time to see changes in a child's condition. Remember that even when you dramatically reduce the level of acid that an asthmatic child is exposed to, it may take weeks for the inflammation in the lungs to settle down, so patience is key, and often treating and waiting is enough to get the wheezing child significant relief.

What about asthmatic children who have no obvious symptoms of reflux? If their airway disease doesn't respond to therapy in a way that's expected by their physician, reflux should always be entertained. This is a great situation for a pH probe because it allows us to quantitate a child's reflux and potentially correlate it with things during the day such as sleeping, exercising, and eating. Though pH probes aren't perfect, children with the most severe lung disease due to reflux will usually show some signs by pH probe. Children with asthma and known reflux whose disease fails to respond to medical therapy may be candidates for fundoplication.

Dental Erosions—The Smoking Gun of Pediatric Reflux

Another difference between babies and older children is the presence of teeth. And just like acid can damage the lining of the esophagus, it can damage the enamel of a child's teeth. Typically, the dental findings of reflux involve the sides of the teeth closest to the tongue, although any part of the enamel can be damaged. Pediatric dentists are becoming more aware of the dental signs of reflux and referring children for evaluation. The solution to dental enamel loss from acid reflux is to fix the reflux, but dentists can sometimes use special sealants to minimize damage.

Barrett's Esophagus:
Can My Child Get Esophageal Cancer?

Parents can't help but think of their kids as little adults. In doing so, we think of their problems as being like the problems that plague us. Chest pain from reflux, for example, is considered a heart attack until proven otherwise. Hemorrhoids, though extremely rare in children, top the parental list of concerns when toddlers experience rectal bleeding. And with all of the direct-to-consumer marketing for acid-suppression medications, parents seem to be asking more and more about esophageal cancer when it looks like their child's reflux is becoming chronic.

I want to nip this in the bud by letting you know that

esophageal cancer from reflux in children fits into the exquis-
itely rare category, probably along the lines of getting hit by
lightning. But because you asked, you might as well be informed about some of the things that you may have heard.
Let's look at the facts—or better, at what we know and what we
don't know.

Years of acid exposure can put the esophagus at risk for dangerous changes that can include cancer. When these changes
begin to take place, they evolve through a fairly predictable sequence. One of the earliest signs that things are headed in the
wrong direction is the development of a finding called *Barrett's
esophagus*, a characteristic change in the cells found in the lining of the esophagus. Through an endoscope, it looks like
salmon-colored patches. Why some people develop Barrett's
esophagus isn't known, but it's believed to be caused by the
same factors that cause reflux. And though anyone can get Barrett's, it's three to five times more common in those with reflux.
It's much more common in men than in women, and if you're
a Caucasian male, you're at the highest risk.

Barrett's esophagus is important because it precedes a particular kind of cancer—esophageal adenocarcinoma. For adults
with Barrett's, the absolute risk of developing esophageal cancer is only about 1%. Esophageal cancer is a particular problem
because it's usually diagnosed late and it's tough to treat.

And what about kids? Barrett's esophagus is so rare in childhood that very little reliable research on the subject exists. In
fact, we don't have a very good idea of its prevalence in children. But those of us who happen to spend much of our time
rooting around the gullets of young kids can attest to the fact
that it's as rare as hen's teeth. The threat of esophageal cancer
shouldn't keep you up at night, but remember that close moni-

toring by a pediatric gastroenterologist is the first step in preventing that infinitely small risk from ever becoming a reality.

A FINAL WORD

As children grow, the problems that they encounter from reflux change. Profound irritability and poor feeding represent the earliest symptoms of reflux, and we have seen that other problems can sometimes follow a child beyond those first several months of life. As I have said several times in this book, care for your child with reflux requires vigilance and close attention on your part. The greatest role that you will play in the caring of your screaming baby is as her advocate. The way you educate yourself, the questions you ask, and your persistence in seeking treatable solutions will set you apart from the parents of past generations. *Colic Solved* may not have given you all of the answers, but it has hopefully served to empower you by helping you to ask all of the right questions.

Our understanding of what makes babies scream is in its infancy. This is one of the first books for parents to suggest that *colic* is a term of the past, and there's a lot more to learn about screaming babies and their reflux. Hopefully, the field of pediatric gastroenterology will advance to the point where this book will serve as amusement for physicians and parents of future generations.

APPENDIX

REFLUX ANATOMY

To understand what's happening in the child with reflux, it's important to understand what happens to food when it is eaten. The upper intestinal tract serves as the starting point in the digestion and absorption of food. It consists of the mouth, esophagus, stomach, and duodenum. The upper intestinal tract also serves as the starting point for reflux. Pay attention because the terms described ahead will serve as a road map when discussing reflux and its causes with your baby's physician.

MOUTH AND PHARYNX

Often overlooked as an important part of digestion, the mouth is where it all begins. Chewing plays a key role in preparing solid food for swallowing. And even before babies have teeth, their saliva contains key enzymes in initiating the breakdown

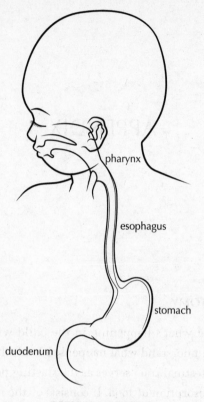

REFLUX ANATOMY

of food. Saliva also contains antacid material that helps protect the swallowing tube from the harmful effects of acid exposure. Once we sense that food is soft enough, it is pushed to the back of the throat, where it enters the pharynx, or the common area where the windpipe and swallowing tube meet. As this occurs, the opening of the windpipe is covered to prevent food from entering the lungs, and food or liquid enters the swallowing tube. Swallowing is a complicated process that involves the coordination of lots of muscles.

FIRST GULPS

The fetus can demonstrate regular swallowing by 16 weeks' gestation. By week 21, a fetus swallows about a half ounce of amniotic fluid every day.

The act of swallowing requires a certain degree of maturation of the nerves and muscles of the mouth and throat. The ability to suck appears at about 32 to 34 weeks of gestation. Babies born more than 2 months premature may not be able to suck and swallow and often need supportive care with tube feeding. And despite the fact that most babies don't have 'em, teeth play a very important role in digestion after the first year of life. Mastication, or chewing, is a critical part of preparing food for early digestion and swallowing. And because they live where reflux can creep, teeth can ultimately be damaged by reflux.

THE ESOPHAGUS—NOT JUST A LAUNDRY CHUTE FOR MILK

The esophagus (swallowing tube) is the tube that connects the pharynx to the stomach. Its job is to bring food from the back of the throat to the stomach. Most parents think of the esophagus as akin to a laundry chute, but it is actually a very complicated organ made up of a complex array of nerves and muscles. (In fact, the number of nerves in the digestive tract approximately equals the number of nerves found in the spinal cord!) These nerves and muscles work together to create waves of squeezing that carry food from the back of the throat to the stomach. These waves are called *peristalsis*. The esophagus can even sense the type of food that comes its way and adjust itself to create different waves for liquid and solid food.

At the bottom of the esophagus there is a circular band of muscles called the *lower esophageal sphincter* (LES). This band of muscles relaxes when food comes to the far end of the esophagus and remains open for about 10 to 12 seconds. Otherwise, it remains closed and serves to keep food from coming into the esophagus once it is in the stomach. Parents like to think of this muscular band as a valve, but it really isn't.

Recognizing that the esophagus is a sensitive, highly innervated organ involved in a very coordinated pattern of squeezing is important because when it gets inflamed or unhappy, it doesn't do its job. As we have learned, an inflamed esophagus that doesn't do its job can create pain, choking, and feeding difficulty in a baby.

STOMACH

Once food is swallowed, its first resting spot is the stomach. While the stomach performs a variety of important digestive functions, its primary job is to break down food into smaller pieces so that nutrients may be absorbed in the intestine. It achieves this through the production of digestive juices and a slow, nearly continuous, squeezing motion.

The stomach juices responsible for this first step in food breakdown consist of hydrochloric acid and an assortment of enzymes that begin to break food down into their most basic elements. We tend to think of the stomach as nothing more than a physiologic garbage disposal, but certain types of fat can be absorbed directly through the lining of the stomach. This is

IT GROWS SO QUICKLY

The esophagus is 8 to 10 centimeters long at birth and doubles in length during the first 2 to 3 years of life.

particularly important because the liver and the pancreas aren't always up to snuff to do the fat absorption necessary for normal growth in babies.

Much as in the esophagus, the squeezing action of the stomach is dependent on the coordination of nerves and muscles to create waves. In fact, the stomach contains a cluster of nerve cells that behave like the pacemaker found in the heart. Every 20 seconds, this cluster of nerves sends out an impulse that begins the process of stomach squeezing. It's this squeezing, along with the exposure to acid, that leads to food breakdown.

In addition to facilitating food breakdown, the squeezing of the stomach helps push food down and out of the stomach for nutrient absorption in the intestine. The rhythmic nerve impulses and squeezing initiated in the stomach move all the way down through the intestine. (For technically oriented readers, these are called *migrating motor complexes*). This is the force that carries food all the way through the digestive system. It all begins in the stomach.

DUODENUM

When food leaves the stomach, it consists of a mushy liquid called *chyme*. Very little nutrient absorption occurs in the stomach. This is the job of the small intestine. Once in the intestine, food is exposed to bile from the liver and enzymes from the pancreas that aid in food breakdown. These digestive enzymes reduce food to its most basic form so that it can be absorbed through the intestinal lining and used for energy and growth. The lining of the small intestine is specially adapted for the transport of nutrients from the bowel into the bloodstream.

The duodenum is the first part of the intestine and begins where the stomach ends. Just as with the esophagus and the stomach, the proper movement of food out of the stomach and through the intestine is dependent on good, healthy contractions. Throughout the length of the small bowel, all useful nutrients and vitamins are absorbed. The small bowel in a baby is approximately 8 feet long and grows as the child grows, achieving its adult length of 22 feet by the time the child is school-age.

COLON

The physiology of the colon has absolutely nothing to do with reflux in kids, but we'll discuss it here as a matter of being complete. Remember that when food, or chyme, reaches the end of the small intestine, the majority of necessary nutrients have been extracted and the remaining mush represents waste material. The job of the colon is to absorb the excess water that remains in this mush. This rescue feature is important in helping babies maintain hydration.

The colon also happens to be the home of millions of different species of bacteria. These bacteria give stool its foul odor and may play a role in the digestion of carbohydrates in babies. Different babies are colonized by different bacteria that are influenced, to some degree, by the types of food they eat. This individual "fingerprint" of bacterial colonization varies from child to child and explains why poops look and smell different. It's interesting to add that when you look at the bacteria colonizing the intestinal tract of a baby, it bears a striking resemblance to that of her parents. Babies get their intestinal bacteria from their parents early in life. The apple doesn't fall far from the tree.

GLOSSARY

aerophagia: The medical word for air swallowing.

antacid: Something that neutralizes acidic solutions.

casein: One of the proteins found in cow's milk. Casein is used as a protein source in some infant formulas. *Casein hydrolysate* formulas are formulas that use broken-down casein as their protein source.

colic: A five-letter word used by physicians when they don't know why a baby is crying.

duodenum: The upper part of the intestinal tract. This is where food goes from the stomach.

EGD: Acronym for *esophagogastroduodenoscopy*, or upper endoscopy. This is the test in which a fiber-optic camera is passed through the mouth and into the stomach and upper small intestine. The lining of the intestine can be examined and biopsied during an EGD.

endoscopy: A general term used to encompass EGD and colonoscopy, the diagnostic studies used for examining the upper and lower intestinal tract.

eosinophil: A type of white blood cell often found in the lining of the intestinal tract in children with protein allergy.

esophagogastroduodenoscopy: *See* **EGD**.

esophagus: The tube that leads from the pharynx to the stomach.

esophagram: An X-ray study in which barium is used to look at the outline of the esophagus. It's used to look for anatomic problems of the esophagus.

fundoplication: A surgical procedure used for the control of gastroesophageal reflux. The procedure involves wrapping the top part of the stomach around the lower part of the esophagus, thereby creating a tighter lower esophageal sphincter and preventing reflux.

fundus: The top part of the stomach.

gastroesophageal reflux disease: The complications and problems arising from the passage of stomach material up and out of the stomach where it doesn't belong.

gastroparesis: The term used to describe weak or absent squeezing of the stomach.

GER: Acronym for *gastroesophageal reflux,* the passage of stomach material up and out of the stomach, where it doesn't belong.

GERD: Acronym for *gastroesophageal reflux disease.*

H₂ blocker: Medications that bind to the stomach's histamine receptors, thereby preventing histamine-stimulated acid secretion.

heartburn: The pain associated with acid reflux. Children can begin to describe heartburn as soon as they're able to talk.

LES: Acronym for *lower esophageal sphincter.*

lower esophageal sphincter: The circular ring of muscles at the bottom of the esophagus that prevents stomach contents from coming back through.

oral aversion: The refusal to feed that evolves when an infant or young child learns to associate feeding or swallowing with some negative sensation such as pain.

parietal cells: The cells in the stomach that make acid.

pH: A scale used to measure the acidity of a liquid. Acids have a low pH, while basic compounds have a high pH.

PPI: Acronym for *proton pump inhibitor.*

Prokinetic medication: A medication used to stimulate squeezing or motility of the intestinal tract.

proton pump inhibitor: A class of drug that reduces the production of stomach acid and heals reflux damage to the esophagus.

pyloric stenosis: A condition of infancy in which the pylorus becomes thickened, thereby preventing stomach contents from entering the intestine. Babies with pyloric stenosis typically present with forceful vomiting at about 1 month of age.

pylorus: The muscle at the bottom of the stomach that helps control what leaves the stomach and how quickly.

reflux: The passage of stomach material proximally out of the stomach where it doesn't belong.

regurgitation: Reflux that comes up to the mouth and sometimes out.

swallow study: A special X-ray study, typically performed by a speech pathologist, in which foods of varying textures and consistencies are given to a patient to see how they are swallowed. Swallow studies are often used to establish that the mechanism of swallowing is safe.

Upper gastrointestinal series: An X-ray study used to evaluate the anatomy of the upper intestinal tract, including the esophagus, stomach, and upper small intestine.

vomiting: The coordinated and reflexive expulsion of stomach contents from the mouth. Vomiting typically involves the coordinated squeezing of the stomach, relaxation of the diaphragm, dilation of the pupils, and salivation.

whey: One of the proteins found in cow's milk.

INDEX

Page numbers in *italics* refer to illustrations.

ABOUT THE AUTHOR

As one of the few pediatric gastroenterologists serving Houston's referral area of nearly 8 million, DR. BRYAN VARTABEDIAN has diagnosed and treated more than 5,000 children with acid reflux disease. He is assistant professor of pediatrics at Baylor College of Medicine in Houston and serves as an attending physician at Texas Children's Hospital, America's largest children's hospital. He is married and the father of an 8-year-old son and a 3-year-old daughter. The issue of reflux disease is of personal interest to Dr. Vartabedian because his daughter suffered during her early months with severe reflux esophagitis. He lives with his family in The Woodlands, Texas.